Pharmaceutical Jurisprudence

Basavaraj K Nanjwade M Pharm, PhD

Professor of Pharmaceutics
Department of Pharmaceutics
KLE University's College of Pharmacy
Belgaum 590010
Karnataka, India

Gurudev M Hiremath M Pharm

Department of Pharmaceutics
KLE University's College of Pharmacy
Belgaum 590010
Karnataka, India

W0193029

CBSPD

CBS Publishers & Distributors Pvt Ltd

New Delhi • Bengaluru • Chennai • Kochi • Kolkata • Lucknow • Mumbai
Hyderabad • Jharkhand • Nagpur • Patna • Pune • Uttarakhand

Disclaimer

Science and technology are constantly changing fields. New research and experience broaden the scope of information and knowledge. The authors have tried their best in giving information available to them while preparing the material for this book. Although, all efforts have been made to ensure optimum accuracy of the material, yet it is quite possible some errors might have been left uncorrected. The publisher, the printer and the authors will not be held responsible for any inadvertent errors or inaccuracies.

PHARMACEUTICAL JURISPRUDENCE

ISBN: 978-93-87085-11-4

Copyright © Publisher

First Edition : 2011

CBS Reprint: 2018, 2019, 2021, 2023

All rights reserved. No part of this book may be reproduced or transmitted in any form or by any means, electronic or mechanical, including photocopying, recording, or any information storage and retrieval system without permission, in written, from the authors and the publisher.

Published by Satish Kumar Jain and produced by Varun Jain for

CBS Publishers & Distributors Pvt Ltd

4819/XI Prahlad Street, 24 Ansari Road, Daryaganj, New Delhi 110 002, India
Ph: 011-23289259, 23266861   Website: www.cbspd.com
                                    e-mail: delhi@cbspd.com
Corporate Office: 204 FIE, Industrial Area, Patparganj, Delhi 110 092, India
Ph: 011-4934 4934   Fax: 011-4934 4935   e-mail: publishing@cbspd.com; publicity@cbspd.com

Branches

- **Bengaluru:** Seema House 2975, 17th Cross, KR Road, Banasankari 2nd Stage, Bengaluru 560 070, Karnataka, India
  Ph: +91-80-26771678/79   Fax: +91-80-26771680   e-mail: bangalore@cbspd.com
- **Chennai:** 7, Subbaraya Street, Shenoy Nagar, Chennai 600 030, Tamil Nadu, India
  Ph: +91-44-26680620, 26681266   Fax: +91-44-42032115   e-mail: chennai@cbspd.com
- **Kochi:** 42/1325, 1326, Power House Road, Opp KSEB, Power House, Ernakulam, Kochi 682 018, India
  Ph: +91-484-4059061–65   Fax: +91-484-4059065   e-mail: kochi@cbspd.com
- **Kolkata:** 147, Hind Ceramics Compound, 1st Floor, Nilgunj Road, Belghoria, Kolkata 700 056, West Bengal, India
  Ph: +91-33-25633055–56   e-mail: kolkata@cbspd.com
- **Lucknow:** Basement, Khushnuma Complex, 7-Meerabai Marg (behind Jawahar Bhawan), Lucknow 226 001, India
  Ph: +91-522-4000032   e-mail: tiwari.lucknow@cbspd.com
- **Mumbai:** PWD Shed. Gala no. 25/26, Ramchandra Bhatt Marg, Next to JJ Hospital Gate no. 2, Opp. Union Bank of India, Noorbaug Mumbai 400 009, Maharashtra, India
  Ph: +91-22-66661880/89   e-mail: mumbai@cbspd.com

Representatives

- **Hyderabad** 0-9885175004 • **Jharkhand** 0-9811541605 • **Nagpur**   0-9421945513
- **Patna**   0-9334159340 • **Pune**   0-9923910676 • **Uttarakhand** 0-9716462459

Printed at Glorious Printers, Jhilmil Industrial Area, Delhi, India

Preface

Jurisprudence is the study of fundamental legal principles including the knowledge of Law. In technical sense it is the science of the first principles of civil laws. Forensic pharmacy (pharmaceutical jurisprudence) Forensic in Latin means a public place, market place or place of assembly for judicial and other business. Some time back, the pharmacy profession was fully controlled in England by Pharmaceutical society of Great Britain and in USA by state laws. The laws in India during this era had superficial references to drugs and medicines. Later in order to control the indiscriminate use of medicines and to legislate the standardization of the preparations and sale of drugs, Government of India in the late Department of Education, Health and Lands, appointed a Drug Enquiry Committee in 1927. Since then many Acts and Laws came into force with various objectives to be meet with, in order to control completely the use of drugs in India.

Though several books are available on the subject, the material in most of them is presented in a diffused form or is highly specialised and discernible to those proficient in the field. The major objective of writing this book is to present the information in a lucid, condensed and cohesive form, to cater specifically the needs of undergraduate students of Pharmacy.

This book consists of 8 chapters. The first chapter introduces to Pharmaceutical Jurisprudence, its Origin & Nature, Scope & Objectives, Evolution of drug laws, various committees etc. It is also gives knowledge about Profession of pharmacy in India, Various Drugs & Pharmaceutical industries in India, Pharmaceutical Education in India and Code of Pharmaceutical Ethics. Chapters 2, 3, 4, 5, 6 & 7 give the features of the Acts thereunder including its objectives, provisions and offences and penalties. Chapters 8 includes salient features of several other Acts such as the Factory act, Shops and Establishment act, Cruelty to animals Act, WTO & GATT, Indian Patents Act etc.

The language and style of this book has been kept simple and lucid to help students to grasp the subject easily. Exhaustive revision questions have been given at the end of each chapter to enable the student to test his comprehension of the subject himself. Efforts have been made to make the book within the constraints of allotted teaching hours for this subject. It is hoped that this book will be well received both by teachers and students.

Author.

Table of Contents

Chapter 4 Medicinal and Toilet Preparations (Excise Duties) Act 1955

Chapter 5 Narcotic Drugs and Psychotropic Substances Act 1985 and A.P.N.D.P.S Rules1986

Chapter 6 Drugs (Prices and control) order 1995

Chapter 7 Drugs and Magic Remedies (objectionable Advertisements) Act 1954 and Rules 1955

Chapter 8 Important Acts

Part A Prevention of cruelty to Animals Act, 1960

Part B AP Shops and establisments Act 1988 and Rule 1990

Part C Factories Act 1948

Part D Generl Agreement on Tariffs and Trade (GATT)

World Trade Organisation (WTO)

Patents Act 1970

Part E Pharmaceutical Policy 2002

Chapter 1

INTRODUCTION

1.1 PHARMACEUTICAL LEGISLATIONS

Jurisprudence: It is the study of fundamental legal principles including the knowledge of Law. In technical sense it is the science of the first principles of civil laws.

Forensic pharmacy (pharmaceutical jurisprudence): Forensic in Latin means a public place, market place or place of assembly for judicial and other business. This signifies that the proposals are decided at the forum or by the public and thus laws are made in the democratic set up. Thus forensic medicine is the application of pharmaceutical knowledge to legal problems.

Act: Legislature makes and approves the Law which are framed by the draftsman. The Act is first set up by the ministry and later the bill is passed by the legislature in the full-fledge statue (expression of will of the legislature). Thus an Indian statue is an Act of the central or state legislatures.

A statute usually consists of the following parts,

1. Date of consent by the president of India.
2. Preamble.
3. Title.
4. Heading.

5.   Marginal notes and punctuations.

6.   Interpretation clauses.

7.   Enacting clauses.

8.   Schedules.

The various legislative instruments and their sub-divisions are as follows.

Instruments	Sub-divisions
Acts	Sections, sub-sections, paragraphs.
Bills	Clause, sub-clause, paragraph.
Orders	Articles, paragraphs, sub-paragraphs.
Regulations	Regulations, paragraphs, sub-paragraphs.
Rules	Rule, paragraphs, sub-paragraphs.
Schedules	Paragraphs, sub-paragraphs.

Schedule: It may contain forms in which powers given under act may be exercised and rights and claims asserted.

ORIGIN AND NATURE

In ancient India wherein synthetic drugs and biological products such as vaccines and sera had not yet evolved, drugs of vegetable, animal. and mineral origin were prepared and utilized. There were very few written laws that time and there was no legal control on pharmacy and medical profession.

Allopathic era started in India around 1840. During this era, most of the allopathic drugs were imported from abroad and some began to be manufactured in India.

During this time "profit rather than service" was the main motive in dealing drugs and medicinal products. Spurious, substandard and adulterate drugs became more common than standard and genuine drugs. Quack medicine and adulterated drugs manufactured in all the parts of the world were supplied to India. There was very common occurrence of offences related to drugs. There was no authority to control such activities.

Except Poison Act, 1919, there was no other law in India that regulated import, manufacture, advertising or sale of drugs. The other laws that had indirect bearing on drugs are as follows,

1. *Indian Panel Code*- Refers to international adulteration.

2. *The Opium Act 1857, 1878*- Refers to cultivation of Poppy and manufacture, possession, transport, export, import and sale of morphine.

3. *The Indian Merchandise Act 1889, 1958*- Refers to misbranding of goods in general.

4. *The Indian Tariff Act 1894 and The Sea Custom Act 1898*- Refers to the levy of custom duty.

5. *The Cantonments Act 1924*- Refers to the entry into any shop and seizure of any medicine which was adulterated.

6. *Dangerous Drug Act 1930.*

These laws had superficial references to drugs and medicines. In the same era, the pharmacy profession was fully controlled in England by Pharmaceutical society of Great Britain and in USA by state laws.

In order to control the indiscriminate use of medicines and to legislate the standardization of the preparations and sale of drugs, Government of India in the late Department of Education, Health and Lands, appointed a Drug Enquiry Committee in 1927 with Col. Sir Ramnath Chopra as its Chairman. Following the committee's report, India Drugs Bill was introduced in the Central Legislature in 1940 and Government of India passed an Act no XXIII of 1940, known as The Drug Act 1940. This is also known as "Preconstituted Act".

SCOPE AND OBJECTIVES

The following pharmaceutical legislation and actions of the Central Government were recommended by Chopra committee.

1. The Drug Act 1940, to regulate the import, manufacture, distribution and sale of drugs. The drug rules 1945, gives effect to the provision of Act.

2. The Pharmacy Act 1948, to regulate the profession and practice of pharmacy, education regulation, prescribe minimum qualification for registration as pharmacist.

3. Drug testing laboratories set up at state and central government.

4. The advisory board- DTAB and DCC have been set up.

5. The manufacturing of Ayurvedic, Siddha, Unani, Tibb and Homeopathic medicines has been brought under Drug and Cosmetic Act.

6. Registration of all drugs and formulations sold in India.

7. An Indian pharmacopoeia has been developed and revised.

8. Ayurvedic pharmacopoeia has been developed.

Drug legislation has the following basic elements

1. General provision:

a) Title.

b) Purpose.

c) Extent.

d) Application of other laws not repealed.

e) Definitions.

2. Specific provisions.

a) Control of Import of drugs.

b) Control of Export of drugs.

c) Control of Manufacture of drugs.

d) Control of Distribution, Storage and Sale of drugs.

e) Control of Advertisement of drugs.

f) Labelling of Drug in General and Specific.

g) Drug Registration and Deregistration.

h) Imposition of Registration Fees.

i) Drugs for Veterinary Use.

j) Drug recall procedures.

k) Scheduling of Drugs.

3. Drug control administration

a) Organisation and functions.

- Central Administrative body.

- Drug Registration Board and Committee.

- Inspectorate services.

- Analytical services.

- Regulatory services.

- Public relations and Consumer affairs Department.

b) Prohibition, offences, penalties and legal procedures.

c) Powers to make Rules and Regulations.

d) Exemption from the provision of the Law.

e) Repeals of other Laws or Regulations.

THE EVOLUTION OF DRUGS LAWS

There are two types of drug laws-

a) Pre-constitution laws.

b) Post constitution laws.

Pre-constitution laws

The laws were passed before independence. In Pre-constitution laws, the state governments are empowered to make changes as their requirements with prior assent of the president.

There is four such type of act-

a)   The Opium Act-1857, 1878.

b)   The Poison Act -1919.

c)   The Dangerous Drug Act- 1930.

d)   The Drug Act- 1940, 1949, 1950, 1951, 1955, 1960, 1962, 1964, 1972, 1982, 1986, 1995.

Post constitution laws

These laws are passed after independence, as per Indian constitution. The state governments are not empowered to make any changes. Such types of act are as follows.

a)   The Pharmacy act- 1948.

b)   The Drug and Magic Remedies (Objectionable Advertisement) Act- 1954.

c)   The Medicinal and Toilet Preparation (Excise Duties) Act- 1955, 1976.

d)   The Drug (Prices Display and Control) Order- 1966, 1969, 1970, 1987, 1995.

e)   Insecticides Act- 1968.

f)   Medicinal Termination of Pregnancy Act- 1971, 1975.

g)   The Narcotic Drugs and Psychotropic Substance Act- 1985.

HEALTH SURVEY AND DEVELOPMENT COMITTEES

1.   **Mudaliar Committee:** The concern of the Health Survey and Planning Committee (Mudaliar Committee 1962) was limited to the development of the health services infrastructure and the health care at the primary level. It felt the growth of infrastructure needed radical transformation and further investment. Another major shift came in the Third Plan (1961-66) when family planning received priority for the first time. Increase in the population became a major worry and was seen as a hurdle to the development process.

Although the broad objective was to bring about progressive improvement in the health of the people by ensuring a certain minimum level of physical well-being and to create conditions favourable for greater efficiency, there was a shift in focus from preventive health services to family planning. During the Fourth Plan (1969-74), efforts were made to provide an effective base for health services in rural areas by strengthening the PHCs. The vertical campaigns against communicable diseases were further intensified.

2. **Bhatia Committee:** Government of India in 1953 appointed a committee under the chairmanship of Major General S.L.Bhatia which is called as Bhatia committee to make comprehensive enquiry into the working of Pharmaceutical industry & to recommend what steps the Government should take to establish it on sound lines in the interest of the country 's health care delivery & economy.

3. **Hathi Committee:** Indian Government has setup Hathi committee under the chairmanship of Jaysukhlal Hathi to take comprehensive look into the drug industry and to enquiry in to the various facts of drugs in India. The report of this committee covered all aspects ranging from licensing, Price control, Imports, role of foreign sector and quality control. It encouraged the development of indigenous industries, It also further controlled price of a large number of drugs in the interest of the consumer.

4. **Bhore committee:** In 1943, Indian Government appointed a committee under the chairmanship of Sir Joseph Bhore to make a survey of existing position of Drug industries in respect to the health care delivery organization in India and to make recommendation for future developments.

Recommendation of Bhore committee

a) Setting up Central Drug Laboratory (CDL).

b) Establishment of all India Pharmaceutical council and provincial Pharmaceutical Council representing the pharmaceutical trade, education.

c) Starting of revised courses of study for:

- Licentiate Pharmacist.

- Pharmaceutical Technologist.

- Graduate Pharmacist.

d) Rigid enforcement of the Drugs and cosmetic act, 1940 throughout the country.

Drug Enquiry Committee: The government of India pursuance to the resolution appointed a committee known as Drug Enquiry Committee with Col.Ramnatha.N.Chopra as its chairman in, 1928.

Recommendation of Chopra Committee

1. A central law to control drug and pharmacy profession.

2. Setting up of testing laboratories in all states to control quality of production of drugs and pharmaceutical and a central laboratory to control the quality of imported drugs and also to act as expert a referee in case of sample sent by local government.

3. Appointment of advisory board to advice the government in making rules to carry out the objectives of the act.

4. Setting up the course for training of pharmacist and prescribe minimum qualification for the registration as the pharmacist.

5. Registration of every pattern and proprietary medicine manufacture in India or imported from outside country.

6. Bringing of crude single drug as well as compounded medicine used in the indigenous system of treatment under control.

7. Development of the drug industry in India.

8. Gradual reduction of manufacturing in medical stores.

9. Completion of an Indian Pharmacopoeia.

NEW DRUG POLICY

In September 1994, a new drug policy was announced with an intension of liberalization of economy and to attract foreign capital. This policy was modified in 1986.

Features of new drug policy

1. Abolished licensing requirements except-

    *   Bulk drugs Vit-B1, Vit-B6, folic acid, tetracycline, oxytetracycline.

    *   Bulk drug produced by the use of recombinant DNA technology.

    *   Bulk drug requiring use of nucleic acids.

2. Replaces two lists of 142 price controlled drugs by single list of 76 drugs.

3. Set up National Drug Authority.

4. A National Pharmaceutical Pricing Authority set up for fixing and revising drug prices.

5. Exemption from price control for ten years for a new drug produced with indigenous technology,

6. Provides incentive for Pharmaceutical Research and Development,

7. Provides for automatic approval of Foreign Technology agreement.

8. Foreign equity ceiling raise from 40% to 50%.

PHARMACY AS A HEALTH CARE SYSTEM

Pharmacy renders a health service and pharmacists are the health professionals. Pharmacists are useful in health services as follows,

1. Preservation of drugs.

2. Prescription adherence.

3. Drug monitoring.

4. Selection of essential drugs.

5. Clinical pharmacological research.

6. Provide information and educate the patients regarding proper use of drugs.

7.   Research and development.

PROFESSION OF PHARMACY IN INDIA

In India the profession of pharmacy consists of,

1.   Teaching profession.

2.   Industrial and manufacturing pharmacist.

3.   Hospital pharmacist.

4.   Licensing and control authority.

5.   Community pharmacist (retail pharmacist).

The first institute of pharmacy was started in Banaras Hindu University in 1932 by Professor M.L. Schroff. Presently many institutions in India provides different courses like-

• Diploma in pharmacy (D.Pharm).

• Bachelor of pharmacy (B.Pharm).

• Master of pharmacy (M.Pharm).

• Doctor of philosophy (Ph.D).

A National Institute for Pharmacy Education and Regulation (NIPER) has been set up by government of India in Mohali, Punjab to improve the quality of teaching and research.

A grant-in-aid institute, by government of Gujarat by B.V.Patel Pharmaceutical Education and Research Development Centre (B.V.Patel PERD) has been set up at Sarkhej-Gandhinagar highway, Ahemdabad.

1.2 DRUGS AND PHARMACEUTICAL INDUSTRY

DRUGS

A drug is "a chemical" substance used in the treatment, cure, prevention, or diagnosis of disease or used to otherwise enhance physical or mental well-being." Drugs may be prescribed for a limited duration, or on a regular basis for chronic disorders.

When drug is absorbed into the body of a living organism, alters normal bodily function. There is no single, precise definition, as there are different meanings in drug control law, government regulations, medicine, and colloquial usage.

Recreational drugs are chemical substances that affect the central nervous system, such as opioids or hallucinogens. They may be used for perceived beneficial effects on perception, consciousness, personality, and behavior. Some drugs can cause addiction and habituation.

A medication or medicine is a drug taken to cure and/or ameliorate any symptoms of an illness or medical condition, or may be used as medicine that has future benefits but does not treat any existing or pre-existing diseases or symptoms.

Drugs are usually distinguished from endogenous biochemicals by being introduced from outside the organism. For example, insulin is a hormone that is synthesized in the body; it is called a hormone when it is synthesized by the pancreas inside the body, but if it is introduced into the body from outside, it is called a drug.

Many natural substances such as beers, wines, and some mushrooms, blur the line between food and drugs, as when ingested they affect the functioning of both mind and body.

Drugs can be administered in a number of ways:

1.   Bolus, a substance into the stomach to dissolve slowly.

2.   Inhaled, (breathed into the lungs), as an aerosol or dry powder.

3.   Injected as a solution, suspension or emulsion, either: intramuscular, intravenous, intraperitoneal, intraosseous.

4.   Insufflations, or snorted into the nose.

5.   Orally, as a liquid or solid, that is absorbed through the intestine.

6.   Rectally as a suppository, that is absorbed by the rectum or colon.

7.   Sublingually, diffusing into the blood through tissues under the tongue.

8.   Topically, usually as a cream or ointment. A drug administered in this manner may be given to act locally or systemically.

9.   Vaginally as a suppository, primarily to treat vaginal infections.

CLASSIFICATION OF DRUGS

Medications can be classified in various ways, such as by chemical properties, mode or route of administration, biological system affected, or therapeutic effects. An elaborate and widely used classification system is the Anatomical Therapeutic Chemical Classification System (ATC system). The World Health Organization keeps a list of essential medicines.

A sampling of classes of medicine includes:

1.   Antipyretics: reducing fever (pyrexia/pyresis)

2.   Analgesics: reducing pain (painkillers)

3.   Antimalarial drugs: treating malaria

4.   Antibiotics: inhibiting germ growth

5.   Antiseptics: prevention   of   germ   growth ear burns, cuts and wounds.

The table below gives a list of drugs and the systems of the body on which it is effective.

Sl no	System/Organ	Classes of Drugs
1.	Digestive system	Antacids, H2 receptor antagonist, Laxatives, Antispasmodic, Antidiarrhoeals etc.
2.	Cardiovascular system	Beta-blockers, Calcium channel blockers, diuretics, Antiarrythmics, Antianginals etc.
3.	Central nervous system	Hypnotics, Anaesthetics, Antipsychotics, Antidepressants, Anticonvulsants, Anxiolytics etc
4.	Musculo-skeletal disorders	NSAIDs, Muscle Relaxants, Neuromuscular drugs, and Anticholinesterases
5.	Occular system	NSAIDs, Corticosteroids, Mast Cell Inhibitors, Miotics, Parasympathomimetics
6.	Respiratory system	Bronchodilators, NSAIDs, AntiAllergics, Antitussives, Mucolytics, Decongestants Corticosteroids, Beta2-adrenergic agonists, Anticholinergics, Steroids etc.
7.	Endocrine system	Androgens, Antiandrogens, Gonadotropin, Corticosteroids, Human Growth Hormone etc
8.	Reproductive system or urinary system	Antifungal, Alkalising Agents, Quinolones, Antibitcs, Cholinergics, Anticholinergics, Anticholinesterases, Antispasmodics, 5-alpha reductase inhibitor

PHARMACEUTICAL INDUSTRY

The list of various pharmaceutical industries in India is given in the table below

Slno	Names
1	Amrutanjan Healthcare Limited
2	Aventis Pharma
3	Biocon
4	Cadila Healthcare
5	Cipla
6	Dabur
7	Dr. Reddy's Laboratories
8	GlaxoSmithKline Pharmaceuticals Ltd
9.	Glenmark Pharmaceuticals
10	Hamdard (Wakf) Laboratories
11	Hindustan Antibiotics Limited
12	Lupin Ltd.
13	Medisys Biotech
14	Nectar Lifesciences
15	Opium and Alkaloid Works
16	Piramal Healthcare
17	Ranbaxy Laboratories
18	Strides Arcolab
19	Sun Pharmaceutical
20	Torrent Pharmaceuticals
21	Unichem Laboratories
22	Wockhardt
23	Zandu Realty
24	Panacea Biotec

1.3 PHARMACEUTICAL EDUCATION

INTRODUCTION

Pharmacy education in India, both at the BPharm and MPharm levels, is taught as an industry- and product oriented profession with a focus on the basic sciences. During the past decade, pharmacy education has expanded significantly in terms of number of institutions offering pharmacy program at various levels. However, pharmacy education in India continues to be one of the last options for students aspiring to a university degree. The pharmacists with a BPharm or MPharm generally seek avenues other than pharmacy practice. These pharmacists prefer placements in production, regulatory affairs, management and/ or quality assurance, and marketing with the pharmaceutical industry. Only small numbers of these graduates and postgraduates opt to work in community and institutional pharmacies. In India, diploma holders (DPharm holders) are practicing pharmacists in the global sense as they engage in community or institution pharmacy practice.

A specialized MPharm in pharmacy practice program launched in the 1990s failed to create employment opportunities in practice areas for these postgraduates. The main change that is currently affecting pharmacy practice is the introduction of the PharmD program in India. One thousand four hundred ten students have enrolled in 47 colleges (mostly private sector) localized in a small geographical part (South India) of India. Going by the experience of socioeconomic status of our country, this steep increase in the required study period from the 2-year DPharm to the 6-year PharmD for producing practicing pharmacists raises issues of PharmD-trained pharmacists who seems to be "unavailable" to serve for India.

EDUCATIONAL PROGRAMS

A variety of pharmacy degree programs are offered in India: diploma in pharmacy (DPharm), bachelor of pharmacy (BPharm), master of pharmacy (MPharm), master of science in pharmacy MS(Pharm) and master of technology in pharmacy MTech (Pharm), doctor of pharmacy (PharmD), and doctor of philosophy in pharmacy (PhD). The entry point, for DPharm, BPharm, and PharmD programs is 12 years of formal education in the sciences. The DPharm program requires a minimum of 2 years of didactic coursework followed by 500 hours of required practical training anticipated to be completed within 3 months in either a hospital or community setting. The BPharm involves 4 years of study in colleges affiliated with universities or in a university department. Students holding a BPharm degree can earn an MPharm degree in 2 years, of which the second year is devoted to research leading to a dissertation in any pharmaceutical discipline, for instance pharmaceutics, pharmacology, pharmaceutical chemistry, or pharmacognosy. Recently, MPharm programs on industrial pharmacy, quality assurance, and pharmaceutical biotechnology have been introduced. To train the graduate pharmacist to provide clinical-oriented services, the MPharm program in pharmacy practice was introduced at Jagadguru Sri Shivaratreeswara (JSS) College of pharmacy at Mysore in 1996 and at Ooty in 1997. There are 6 National Institutes of Pharmaceutical Education and Research (NIPERs) in India offering MS(Pharm), MTech(Pharm), and higher-level degrees. The NIPERs were created with the vision of providing excellence in pharmacy and pharmacy-related education. Students with an MPharm degree in any discipline can work toward a PhD with an additional minimum 3 years of study and research. The PharmD program constitutes 6 years of full-time study. The PharmD (post-baccalaureate) program is a 3-year program. The PharmD program was introduced in 2008 with the aim of producing pharmacists who had undergone extensive training in practice sites and could provide pharmaceutical care to patients.

GROWTH OF PHARMACY EDUCATION

Prior to mid 1980s, the growth of publicly funded institutions of higher education (including pharmacy institutions) was very slow. Until early 1980s, there were 11 universities and 26 colleges offering pharmacy education at the bachelor's and master's levels. In addition, there was at least 1 government school in every Indian state offering the DPharm program. Since the late 1980s, due to rapid industrialization in the pharmaceutical sector, privatization, and economic growth, pharmacy education has been developing faster in India than anywhere in the world. In 2007, there were 854 institutions that admitted more than 52,000 students to the BPharm degree program and 583 institutions that trained more than 34,000 students in the DPharm degree program. Most of the institutions, however, are privately funded colleges or privately funded universities. The private sector, which accounted for about 10% of the students admitted in the 1980s, now accounts for 91% of all pharmacy students admitted.

While there are a large number of DPharm and BPharm graduates each year, the number of students that has graduated in any state varies widely. A large number of privately funded institutions are located in states like Tamilnadu, Karnataka, Andhra Pradesh, Maharasthra, and Gujrat. In Tamilnadu, around 45 colleges and universities educate approximately 2,960 DPharm and 2590 BPharm graduates per year (within a total state population of about 64 million).

ADMISSION CRITERIA

Entry qualifications for pharmacy programs vary across and within states, and most significantly, between private and public institutions. Entry requirements also vary depending on the degree program. The majority of privately funded institutions do not have a direct formal application processes. There is no centralized data repository to indicate the number of applicants to private and public institutions in India.

DPharm Program

In India, higher secondary study is concluded by a terminal examination, the higher secondary examination, at the end of 12 years. Admission to the first year DPharm program in any government college is based on performance on the higher secondary examination. However, private colleges have their own admission procedures that comply with the education regulations of the PCI. Students generally may choose to undertake the DPharm program as their second or third choice, having been unable to obtain a place at the college in another degree program that was their first choice. The DPharm curriculum is framed through the education regulations of the Pharmacy Act. The present education regulations framed way back in 1991 (ER91). The curriculum is the same throughout the country. In the 1990s, the efforts of the pharmacy council of India for upgrading the minimum qualification for registration from DPharm to BPharm failed due to lack of consensus.

BPharm Program

Admission to the first-year BPharm program is made directly from higher secondary school on the basis of marks obtained in the higher secondary examination or on the basis of a merit list rank prepared based on scores on an entrance examination administered by a state or individual institution. Administering an entrance examination as an admissions requirement is used mainly by public institutions. For example, admission to the first-year BPharm of Banaras Hindu University (BHU) is made through the joint entrance examination (JEE) conducted by Indian Institutions of Technology (IITs), a group of 13 autonomous engineering and technology-oriented public institutes of higher education established and declared as institutes of national importance by the government of India. The selected students opt for more rewarding bachelor of technology (BTech) programs; therefore, most of the 40 seats open in the BPharm program at BHU remain vacant. The practice regarding preparing a merit list of applicants also differs. Some states and institutions place emphasis on entrance examination scores and use this as the only criterion in the selection process. A few private universities and at least 1 Indian state (Tamilnadu) have abandoned entrance examinations and use grades scored in the higher secondary examination instead. Many government institutions adopt a middle ground and use a combination of grades and entrance examination scores in their selection process. The merit list rank preparation or the entrance examination conduction for admission to the first-year BPharm and bachelor of engineering programs is undertaken jointly in all states except Tamilnadu and Karnataka, where it is combined with the medical degree programs. In general, applicants who rank lower on the list enter a BPharm program. In 2008, more than 35,000 students completed an entrance examination in WestBengal, a northeastern Indian state. The 25,000 students who ranked highest on the list chose to enter engineering programs, while students below this rank selected BPharm programs in private institutions. There were reports in 2008 that institutions were having difficulty attracting suitable candidates to fill openings in their pharmacy programs.

The table below gives the first 10 Pharmacy Colleges/Universities Offering Degree Programs in India.

Year of Inception	Colleges Or Universities	Degree Offered
1937	Department of Pharmaceutical Engineering,Institute of Technology, Banaras HinduUniversity, Varanasi	BPharm, MPharm, PhD
1944	University Institute of PharmaceuticalSciences, Panjab University, Chandigarh	BPharm, MPharm, PhD
1947	L. M. College of Pharmacy, Ahmedabad	BPharm, MPharm, PhD
1950	Department of Pharmacy, Madras MedicalCollege, Chennai	BPharm, MPharm
1950	Birla Institute of Science and Technology,Pilani	BPharm, MPharm, PhD
1951	College of Pharmaceutical Sciences, AndhraUniversity, Visakhapatnam	BPharm, MPharm, PhD
1952	Department of Pharmaceutical Sciences,Dr. H.S. Gour University, Sagaur	BPharm, MPharm, PhD
1956	Department of Pharmaceutical Sciences,Nagpur University, Nagpur	BPharm, MPharm, PhD
1958	Pharmaceutical Department, UniversityInstitute of Chemical Technology,Mumbai University, Mumbai	BPharmSci, MPharmSci, PhD (Tech)
1963	Department of PharmaceuticalTechnology, Jadavpur University, Kolkata	BPharm, MPharm, PhD

MPharm Program

The criterion for entry to an MPharm program is academic performance in the BPharm or an entrance test or both. Currently, there is more demand for the MPharm program than the availability of places in the country. An important criterion, a high Graduate Aptitude Test for Engineering (GATE) score, qualifies a student to receive government scholarship during the period of their MPharm study. This criterion is optional for admission to the first-year MPharm program. However, many public institutions require both past academic performance and GATE score for application to the MPharm program.

PharmD Program

Admission to a PharmD degree program is on the basis of successful completion of the higher secondary examination or the DPharm program. Passing the higher secondary examination with physics, chemistry, and biology or mathematics entitles a student to enter the PharmD program. BPharm degree holders can join the PharmD program in the fourth year.

The table below gives the first 10 Pharmacy Colleges/Universities Offering Degree Programs in India.

CURRICULUM

Curriculum change can be undertaken by central government notification through an amendment of the Pharmacy Act. The basic pharmacy courses of the program consist of mostly old and outdated concepts with many unnecessary topics that are of little practical value. The Pharmaceutics I practical subject is devoted to preparations of aromatic waters, iodine and other simple solutions, tinctures, extracts, and spirits among others. The Pharmaceutics II practical devotes 100 hours to learning at least 100 prescription products and their compounding and dispensing methods, and covers mixture, divided powders, liniments, and various incompatibilities in prescription products. All of these topics are of little relevance in an era where manufactured ready-to-dispense medicines are widely used and accepted.

The orientation of the pharmacist has changed from the product to the patient. The expansion of the role of pharmacists received an important boost in 1990, when Helper and Strand coined the term pharmaceutical care. Pharmaceutical care is the responsible provision of drug therapy for the purpose of achieving definite outcomes that improve the patient's quality of life. Approximately 30,000 students receive DPharm degree each year and enter the profession without being taught pharmaceutical care concepts and many other areas of contemporary pharmacy.

There is no standardized BPharm curriculum and it varies across the universities that offer this degree. It is industry and product oriented. The vast majority of pharmacy colleges offering education are away from practice sites and there is no compulsory training in a practice site. Unlike other countries, the curricular revision and innovation in India have not received adequate attention. The BPharm program of most of the Indian universities includes a mix of basic science (such as mathematics, physical chemistry, inorganic chemistry, and organic chemistry), advanced chemistry and analysis (such as biochemistry, medicinal chemistry, and analytical chemistry) and basic pharmacy (such as pharmaceutics, pharmacology, pharmacognosy, and pharmacy law). The curriculum has 18 laboratory components (82% of theory course work). In addition, it devotes around 40% for chemistry and analysis related subjects. The curriculum does not include coursework in the behavioral and social sciences, and health care policy.

The MPharm degree program requires an additional 2 years of study after a BPharm degree (a total of 6 years of pharmacy study). TheMPharm degree is offered in many disciplines such as pharmaceutics, and pharmacology. The curriculum is divided into 2 parts. The first part consists of 1 year of didactic course work (both theory and laboratory) and the second part involves completing a research project under the supervision of a pharmacy faculty member in a chosen discipline. Students who pursue an MPharm in industrial pharmacy may undertake research projects in pharmaceutical industries during their second year of the curriculum. An industrial expert is responsible for part of the research, serving as the student's co-supervisor.

An MPharm degree in pharmacy practice/clinical pharmacy was started in 1996 with the aim of training the postgraduate pharmacy students in patient-oriented service. Students of such MPharm programs undertake their second- year research projects in either a hospital or community setting. There are 14 colleges, mostly located in South India, that offer the MPharm degree in pharmacy practice. However, most of the BPharm graduates are not attracted to this clinically oriented MPharm program The deficiencies of the program are analyzed in a letter published in the Journal which explains that postgraduates with an MPharm in clinical pharmacy cannot opt to work as clinical pharmacists in Indian hospitals, as the value of clinical pharmacy services is not recognized, and the current regulatory framework does not yet recognize the need for clinical pharmacists at the national level.

REGULATIONS AND QUALITY ISSUES

Pharmacy education in India is regulated by 2 organizations: the Pharmacy Council of India (PCI), under the Pharmacy Act of 1948, and the All India Council for Technical Education (AICTE), which was established under the AICTE Act of 1987. As mentioned previously, the PCI makes regulations regarding the minimum standard of education required for qualification as a pharmacist. It is responsible for registration of persons fulfilling the prescribed eligibility criteria (minimum DPharm) and issuing a license permitting them to practice in an Indian state. Registration activity is decentralized and the state pharmacy councils are responsible for registering pharmacists in their respective states. Thus, the PCI regulates the DPharm program and the recently introduced PharmD program. The BPharm program needs to be recognized by the PCI for the qualifications to be accepted for registration purpose only. The PCI has no jurisdiction over MPharm and other higher-level degree programs. Pharmacy education at all levels excluding the PharmD is regulated by the AICTE and all these programs must be approved by it. The AICTE is primarily responsible for planning, formulating, and maintaining norms and standards in technical education, which include pharmacy. Besides the Pharmacy Act, pharmacy practice is also governed by the Drugs and Cosmetics Act of 1940, which stipulates the manufacture, distribution, and sale of drugs. Currently, there are no regulatory body and regulatory control for clinical pharmacy practice.

The AICTE is also responsible for quality assurance of pharmacy programs (DPharm, BPharm and MPharm) through accreditation by National Board of Accreditation (NBA) constituted by the AICTE. However, only 8% of pharmacy programs have been accredited. Accreditation is voluntary and also a stringent process; thus, few institutions have applied for accreditation on their own. The voluntary accreditation seems to serve little purpose for any of its stakeholders. Unlike other countries, the current regulations do not require any continuing education to maintain licensure once they are conferred. In addition, registered pharmacists do not have any established norms on competencies or standards of services. There is no categorization of practicing and non-practicing pharmacists.

EMPLOYMENT

The DPharm program was developed and designed to train students to serve as institutional and community pharmacists. Pharmacists with a DPharm degree have the opportunity to join a hospital (government or private) or community pharmacy (mostly private). The majority of diploma-trained pharmacists choose to work in government hospitals rather than private hospitals or pharmacies. They are also considered for placements in the pharmaceutical industry. The salary of pharmacists in government positions is lower than the salaries of similarly qualified health professionals (nurses, diagnostic technicians, and radiographers) and pharmacists in privately owned community pharmacies are always underpaid. In the recently accepted Indian government's sixth pay commission recommendations, practicing pharmacists have been placed in the lowest band and structure, along with other nontechnical persons. The vast majority of pharmacists with a BPharm degree normally seek positions (such as production, quality control, and marketing) with the thriving pharmaceutical industries in which services are well defined and industrial pharmacists are well remunerated. They also have the opportunity to be appointed to drug regulatory agencies or quality control laboratories by the state or central government. MPharm degree holders in any discipline including an MPharm in clinical pharmacy may join industries in any of the above positions. Many MPharm graduates entering the pharmaceutical industry choose positions in areas such as research, formulation development, and clinical trials. Additionally, they have the opportunity to work in the academic area, typically as researchers or faculty members. The demand for pharmacists is further growing with the growth of the pharmaceutical industry in India. Pharmacists with a PhD mainly work in academia and in the research and development section of pharmaceutical industries.

1.4 CODE OF PHARMACEUTICAL ETHICS AND POLICY

INTRODUCTION

Ethics may be defined as 'the code of moral principles or as the science of morals'.

Pharmacists are health professionals who assist individuals in making the best use of medications. This Code, prepared and supported by pharmacists, is intended to state publicly the principles that form the fundamental basis of the roles and responsibilities of pharmacists. These principles, based on moral obligations and virtues, are established to guide pharmacists in relationships with patients, health professionals, and society.

PRINCIPLES OF PHARMACIST

The Code of Ethics sets out the principles that you must follow as a pharmacist or pharmacy technician.

1. *A pharmacist respects the covenantal relationship between the patient and pharmacist.*

    Considering the patient-pharmacist relationship as a covenant means that a pharmacist has moral obligations in response to the gift of trust received from society. In return for this gift, a pharmacist promises to help individuals achieve optimum benefit from their medications, to be committed to their welfare, and to maintain their trust.

2. *A pharmacist promotes the good of every patient in a caring, compassionate, and confidential manner.*

    A pharmacist places concern for the well-being of the patient at the centre of professional practice. In doing so, a pharmacist considers needs stated by the patient as well as those defined by health science. A pharmacist is dedicated to protecting the dignity of the patient.

With a caring attitude and a compassionate spirit, a pharmacist focuses on serving the patient in a private and confidential manner.

3. *A pharmacist respects the autonomy and dignity of each patient.*

A pharmacist promotes the right of self-determination and recognizes individual self-worth by encouraging patients to participate in decisions about their health. A pharmacist communicates with patients in terms that are understandable. In all cases, a pharmacist respects personal and cultural differences among patients.

4. *A pharmacist acts with honesty and integrity in professional relationships.*

A pharmacist has a duty to tell the truth and to act with conviction of conscience. A pharmacist avoids discriminatory practices, behaviour or work conditions that impair professional judgment, and actions that compromise dedication to the best interests of patients.

5. *A pharmacist maintains professional competence.*

A pharmacist has a duty to maintain knowledge and abilities as new medications, devices, and technologies become available and as health information advances.

6. *A pharmacist respects the values and abilities of colleagues and other health professionals.*

When appropriate, a pharmacist asks for the consultation of colleagues or other health professionals or refers the patient. A pharmacist acknowledges that colleagues and other health professionals may differ in the beliefs and values they apply to the care of the patient.

7. *A pharmacist serves individual, community, and societal needs.*

The primary obligation of a pharmacist is to individual patients. However, the obligations of a pharmacist may at times extend beyond the individual to the community and society. In these situations, the pharmacist recognizes the responsibilities that accompany these obligations and acts accordingly.

8. *A pharmacist seeks justice in the distribution of health resources.*

When health resources are allocated, a pharmacist is fair and equitable, balancing the needs of patients and society.

CODE OF CONDUCT

Code of conduct can be divided into different groups as follows.

A. Pharmacist in relation to his job

1. Pharmaceutical services:

   a) A pharmacist should supply required medicines without delay.

   b) A pharmacist should willingly provide emergency supplies at all times.

2. Conduct of drug store:

   a) In preparation, dispensing and supply of medicine, there should not be any error of accidental contamination.

   b) There should be clear indication regarding practice of pharmacy.

   c) There should be a notice stating under which particular scheme dispensing is carried out such as E.S.I.S.

   d) Every drug store should be controlled by the qualified pharmacist.

3. Handling of the prescriptions:

   a) Upon receipt of prescription, pharmacist should not show any type of expression, which creates doubt or fear in the mind of the patient.

   b) If any doubt, the patient should be asked with caution and care in a tactful manner.

   c) Pharmacist has no privilege to add, omit or substitute any ingredient without the consent of prescriber unless emergence or pharmaceutical art is required, which does not cause any chage in therapeutic action.

   d) In the case of incompatibility or over dose, the prescription should be referred back to physician.

e) In refilling the prescription, pharmacist should be totally guided by physician and advice the patients according to the direction of the physician.

f) Pharmacist should not discuss with patients regarding therapeutic efficacy of the prescription.

4. Handling of drugs:

a) Standard quality of drug should be used. Never fill the prescription with spurious, substandard and unethical preparation.

b) Weigh and measure all ingredients correctly and accurately. Visual estimations should be avoided.

c) Pharmacist must be very careful in dealing with poisonous, habit forming and abusive drugs.

5. Apprentice pharmacist:

a) Pharmacist should see that trainees are given full facilities, sufficient technique and skill.

B. Pharmacist in relation to his trade

1. Price structure:

a) Customers should be charged with fair price.

b) Pharmacist should get adequate remuneration as per his knowledge, skill and responsibilities.

2. Fair trade practice:

a) There should not be cut throat competition among pharmacies, by giving price or gift to any physicians.

b) Do not dispense or compound the prescription pertaining to other pharmacy, direct the customer to the right place.

c) Do not copy the labels, trade mark or other signs and symbols of other pharmacies.

3. Purchase of drug:

a) Drug should be purchased from standard, genuine and reputable source.

4. Hawking of drugs:

a) Hawking should not be encouraged.

b) Door to door or self service should not be done.

5. Advertising and displays:

a) No display should be used either on the premises, in the press or elsewhere which may-

- Reflect unfavourable pharmacists collectively, or upon any group or individual.
- Disparage other suppliers or product.
- Show misleading or exaggerated statements.
- Give a guarantee.
- Be an appeal to or fear.
- Offer a prize or scheme.
- Be regarding sexual weakness, premature ageing etc.

C. Pharmacist in relation to medical profession

1. Limitation of professional activities:

a) Under no circumstances, pharmacist should take to medical practice. He can only render first aid emergences.

b) Never recommend particular physician unless asked.

2. Commission agreements:

a) There should not be any secret contract with any physician for recommendation of particular drug store.

3. Liaison with public:

a) Pharmacist is a liaison between physician and people, so he himself should be knowledgeable.

b) Pharmacist should never disclose any information to any third party.

c) He should have confidence.

D. Pharmacist in relation to his profession

1. Professional vigilance:

   a) Pharmacist should himself abide the laws and it's his duty to make others also to fulfil the provision of the laws.

   b) Pharmacist has to disclose the names those who are not fulfilling the provisions of the laws.

   c) Pharmacist has to extend help to a fellow pharmacist with respect to legitimate need, scientific or technical.

2. Law-abiding citizen:

   a) Pharmacist must have fair knowledge of the laws pertaining to food, drug, pharmacy, health and sanitation.

3. Relationships with professional organisation:

   a) Pharmacist should be the member of such organisation.

4. Manner and properness:

   a) Pharmacist should act mannerly and properly on pharmaceutical profession.

OATH OF A PHARMACIST

I promise to do all that I can to protect and improve the physical and moral wellbeing of society, holding the health and safety of my community above other considerations. I shall uphold the loss and standards governing my profession avoiding all forms of misrepresentations and I shall safeguard the distribution of medicinal and potent substance.

Knowledge gained about patients, I shall hold in confidence and never disclose unless compelled to do so by law.

I shall try hard to perfect and enlarge my knowledge to contribute the advancement of pharmacy in the public health.

I furthermore promise to maintain my honour in all transactions and by my conduct never bring discredit to myself or to my profession or to do anything to lessen the trust put in my professional friend and colleagues.

May I prosper and live long in favour as I keep an hold to his, my oath, but if I violate these sacred promises, may the reverse be my lot.

REVIEW QUESTIONS

ESSAY QUESTIONS

1. Write a note on origin and nature of Pharmaceutical Legislation in India.

2. Explain the scopes and objectives of Pharmaceutical Legislation in India.

3. Write a note on Health Survey and Development committees.

4. Write a note on Drugs and Pharmaceutical Industries in India.

5. Write a note on Pharmaceutical education in India.

6. A brief account on the Principles of Pharmacist as mentioned in the Code of Pharmaceutical Ethics.

SHORT QUESTIONS

1. Define the following.
   a) Jurisprudence.
   b) Forensic pharmacy.
   c) Act.
   d) Schedule.
   e) Ethics.

2. Write a note on Evolution of Drug laws.

3. What is Drug Enquiry Committee? Explain in brief.

4. Give a brief account on New Drug Policy.

5. Write a note on Pharmacy as a Health care system.

6. Write a note on Profession of Pharmacy in India.

7. Write a note on Pharmacist in relation to his job.

8. Write a note on Pharmacist in relation to his trade.

9. Write a note on Pharmacist in relation to medical profession.

10. Write a note on Pharmacist in relation to his profession.

11. Write a note on Pharmacist Oath.

Chapter 2

PHARMACY ACT 1948

2.1 INTRODUCTION

An Act to regulate the profession of pharmacy. It is expedient to make better provision for the regulation of the profession and practise of pharmacy and for that purpose to constitute Pharmacy Councils.

This Act may be called the Pharmacy Act, 1948. It extends to the whole of India except the State of Jammu and Kashmir. It shall come into force at once.

The pharmacy act was passed in 1948 and then subsequently amended as follows,

- Pharmacy (amendment) Act, 1959
- Pharmacy (amendment) Act, 1976
- Pharmacy (amendment) Act, 1981

OBJECTIVES

The main objectives of the Act are as follows,

1. Restoration of the pharmacy profession in its due place in the health service.
2. Raising the status of pharmacy profession in India.
3. To regulate the practice of pharmacy in India.
4. To provide uniform education and training throughout India.

5. To maintain control over persons entering the profession of pharmacy.

DEFINITIONS

1. *Registered medical practitioners (R.M.P):* A person holding a qualification granted by an authority notified under Section 3 of the Indian Medical Degrees Act or specified in the schedules to the Indian Medical Council Act.

2. *Registered pharmacist:* A person whose name is for the time-being entered in the register of the state in which he or she is for the time-being residing or carrying on his profession or business of pharmacy.

3. *Central Register*: Means the register of pharmacists maintained by the Central Council under section 15 A.

4. *Executive Committee*: Means the Executive Committee of the Central Council or of the State Council, as the context may require.

5. *Central Council*: Means the Pharmacy Council of India constituted under section 3.

6. *State Council:* means a State Council of Pharmacy constituted under section 19, and includes a Joint State Council of Pharmacy constituted in accordance with an agreement under section 20.

2.2 PHARMACY COUNCIL IN INDIA

In order to meet the above objectives Central Council of Pharmacy (Pharmacy Council of India – P.C.I) and Provisional (State) Pharmacy Council (S.P.C) were constituted.

A.   PHARMACY COUNCIL OF INDIA (P.C.I)

The P.C.I is constituted by the central government and first P.C.I was constituted in 1949. The council is reconstituted every 5 years. P.C.I consists of 3 different types of members.

1. Elected members.

2. Nominated members.

3. Ex-officio members.

ELECTED MEMBERS

1. Six members, elected by university grants commission from amongst the teaching staff of a university or college granting a degree or diploma in pharmacy.

Amongst these, three should be at least a teacher each of pharmacy, pharmaceutical chemistry, pharmacognosy and pharmacology.

2. One member, elected by Medical Council of India.

3. One member, elected by state pharmacy council from amongst its members, to represent each state.

NOMINATED MEMBERS

1. Six members, nominated by the central government, of whom, at least four should possess a degree or diploma in pharmacy and should be engaged in the practice of pharmacy or pharmaceutical chemistry.

2. A representative of U.G.C and a representative of A.I.C.T.E.

3. One member, nominated by each state government/ Union Territory.

EX-OFFICIO MEMBERS

1. The Director General of Health Service.

2. The Director of Central Drug Laboratory.

3. The Drug Controller of India.

The President and the Vice-president of the council are elected by the Council members from its own members.

The Council may appoint a Registrar (who shall act as secretary or as a treasure too) and other officers and servants as necessary.

The Central Council constitutes an Executive Committee consisting of,

1. President (chairman).

2. Vice-president (Ex-officio)

3. Five other members elected by Central Council from its members.

President, Vice-president and nominated members hold office for a period not exceeding 5 years.

A nominated or elected member are considered to have vacated his seat if he remains absent for three consecutive meetings.

FUNCTIONS OF P.C.I

The following are the function of P.C.I.

Education Regulations

1. Subject to the provisions of this section, the Central Council may, subject to the approval of the Central Government, make regulations, to be called the Education Regulations, prescribing the minimum standard of education required for qualification as a pharmacist.

2. In particular and without prejudice to the generality of the foregoing power, the Education Regulations may prescribe-

    a)   The nature and period of study and of practical training to be undertaken before admission to an examination.

    b)   The equipment and facilities to be provided for students undergoing approved courses of study.

    c)   The subjects of examination and the standards therein to be attained.

    d)   Any other conditions of admission to examinations.

3. Copies of the draft of the Education Regulations and of all subsequent, amendments thereof shall be furnished by the Central Council to all State Governments, and the Central Council shall

before submitting the Education Regulations or any amendment thereof, as the case may be, to the Central Government for approval under sub-section (1) take into consideration the comments of any State Government received within three months from the furnishing of the copies as aforesaid.

4. The Education Regulations shall be published in the Official Gazette and in such other manner as the Central Council may direct.

5. The Executive Committee shall from time to time report to the Central Council on the efficacy of the Education Regulations and may recommend to the Central Council such amendments thereof as it may think fit.

Application of Education Regulations to States

At any time after the constitution of the State Council and after consultation with the State Council, the State Government may, by notification in the Official Gazette, declare that the Education Regulations shall take effect in the State.

Provided that where no such declaration has been made, the Education Regulations shall take effect in the State on the expiry of three years from the date of the constitution of the State Council.

Approved courses of study and examinations

1. Any authority in a State which conducts a course of study for pharmacists may apply to the Central Council for approval of the course, and the Central Council, if satisfied, after such enquiry as it thinks fit to make, that the said course of study is in conformity with the Education Regulations, shall declare the said course of study to be an approved course of study for the purpose of admission to an approved examination for pharmacists.

2. Any authority in a State which holds an examination in pharmacy may apply to the Central Council for approval of the examination, and the Central Council, if satisfied, after such enquiry as it thinks fit to make, that the said examination is in conformity with the Education Regulations, shall declare the said examination to be an

approved examination for the purpose of qualifying for registration as a pharmacist under this Act.

3.   Every authority in the State which conducts an approved course of study or holds an approved examination shall furnish such information as the Central Council may, from time to time, require as to the courses of study and training and examination to be undergone, as to the ages at which such courses of study and examination are required to be undergone and generally as to the requisites for such courses of study and examination.

Withdrawal of approval

1.   Where the Executive Committee reports to the Central Council that an approved <u>course</u> of study or an approved examination does not continue to be in conformity with the Education Regulations, the Central Council shall give notice to the authority concerned of its intention to take into consideration the question of withdrawing the declaration of approval accorded to the course of study or examination, as the case may be, and the said authority shall within three months from the receipt of such notice forward to the Central Council through the State Government such representation in the matter as it may wish to make.

2.   After considering any representation which may be received from the authority concerned and any observations thereon which the State Government may think fit to make, the council may declare that the course of study or the examination shall be deemed to be approved only when completed or passed, as the case may be, before a specified date.

Qualifications granted outside the territories to which this Act extends

The Central Council, if it is satisfied that any qualification in pharmacy granted by an authority outside the territories to which this Act extends affords a sufficient guarantee of the requisite skill and knowledge, may declare such qualification to be an approved qualification for the purpose of qualifying for registration under this Act, and may for reasons appearing to it sufficient at any time declare that such qualification shall be deemed to be approved only when granted before or after a specified date:

Provided that no person other than a (citizen of India) possessing such qualification shall be deemed to be qualified for registration unless by the law and practice of the State or Country in which the qualification is granted, persons of Indian origin holding such qualification are permitted to enter and practise the profession of pharmacy.

Mode of declarations

All declarations under section 12, section 13 or section 14 shall be made by resolution passed at a meeting of the Central Council, and shall have effect as soon as they are published in the Official Gazette.

The Central Register

1. The Central Council shall cause to be maintained in the prescribed manner a register of pharmacists to be known as the Central Register, which shall contain the names of all persons for the time being entered in the register for a State.

2. Each State Council shall supply to the Central Council five copies of the register for the State as soon as may be after the first day of April of each year, and the Registrar, of each State Council, shall inform the Central Council, without delay, all additions to, and other amendments in, the Register for the State made from time to time.

3. It shall be the duty of the Registrar of the Central Council to keep the Central Register in accordance with the orders made by the Central Council, and from time to time to revise the Central Register and publish it in the Gazette of India.

4. The Central Register shall be deemed to be public document within the meaning of the Indian Evidence Act, 1872 (1 of 1872) and may be proved by the production of a copy of the Register as published in the Gazette of India.

Registration in the Central Register

The Registrar of the Central Council shall, on receipt of the report of registration of a person in the register for a State, enter his name in the Central Register.

B.   PROVISIONAL PHARMACY COUNCIL

The provisional pharmacy council may be classified as follows,

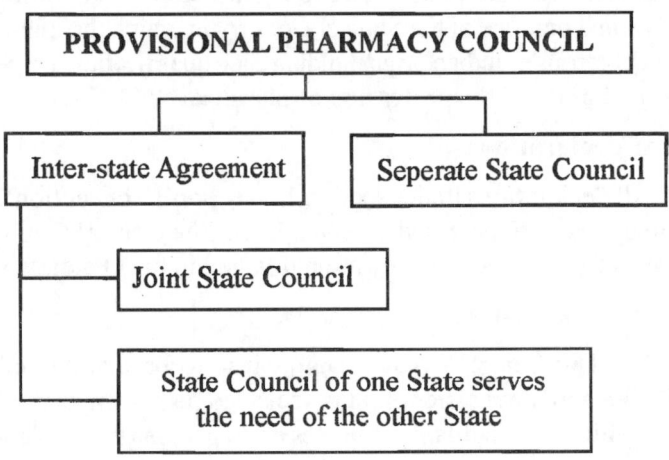

2.3 SEPERATE STATE COUNCIL

Constitution and Composition of State Councils

Except where a Joint State Council is constituted in accordance with an agreement made under section 20, the State Government shall constitute a State Council consisting of the following members, namely-

1. Six members, elected from amongst themselves by registered pharmacists of the State.

2. Five members, of whom at least three shall be persons possessing a prescribed degree or diploma in pharmacy or pharmaceutical chemistry or registered pharmacists, nominated by the State Government.

3. One member elected from amongst themselves by the members of each Medical Council or the Council of Medical Registration of the State, as the case may be;

4. The chief administrative medical officer of the State ex officio or if he is unable to attend any meeting, a person authorized by him in writing to do so.

The officer-in-charge of drugs control organization of the State under the Drugs and Cosmetics Act, 1940, ex officio or if he is unable to attend any meeting, a person authorized by him in writing to do so.

5. The Government Analyst under the Drugs and Cosmetics Act, 1940, ex officio, or where there is more than one, such one as the State Government may appoint in this behalf.

Provided that where an agreement is made under clause (b) of sub-section (1) of section 20, the agreement may provide that the State Council to serve the needs of the other participating States also shall be augmented by not more than two members, of whom at least one shall at all times be a person possessing a prescribed degree or diploma in pharmacy or pharmaceutical chemistry or a registered pharmacist, nominated by the Government of each of the said other participating States, and where the agreement so provides, the composition of the State Council shall be deemed to 'be augmented accordingly.

2.4 INTER-STATE AGREEMENT

1. Two or more State Government may enter into an agreement to be in force for such period and to be subject to renewal for such further periods, if any, as may be specified in the agreement, to provide-

   a) For the constitution of a Joint State Council for all the participating States, or

   b) That the State Council of one State shall serve the needs of the other participating States.

2. In addition to such matters as are in this Act specified, an agreement under this section may-

a)   Provide for the apportionment between the participating State of the expenditure in connection with the State Council or Joint State Council.

b)   Determine which of the participating State Governments shall exercise the several functions of the State Government under this Act, and the references in this Act to the State Government shall be construed accordingly.

c)   Provide for consultation between the participating State Governments either generally or with reference to particular matters arising under this Act.

d)   Make such incidental and ancillary provisions, not inconsistent with this Act, as may be deemed necessary or expedient for giving effect to the agreement.

3. An agreement under this section shall be published in the Official Gazettes of the participating States.

Composition of Joint State Councils

1. A Joint State Council shall consist of the following members, namely-

a.   Such number of members, being not less than three and not more than five as the agreement shall provide elected from amongst themselves by the registered pharmacists of each of the participating States.

b.   Such number of members, being not less than two and not more than four as the agreement shall provide, nominated by each participating State Government.

c.   One member elected from amongst themselves by the members of each Medical Council or the Council of Medical Registration of each participating State as the case may be.

d.   The Chief Administrative Medical Officer of each participating State, ex officio, or if he is unable to attend any meeting, a person authorized by him in writing to do so.

The officer-in-charge of drugs control organization of each participating State under the Drugs and Cosmetics Act, 1940, ex officio, or if he is unable to attend any meeting, a person authorized by him in writing to do so.

e.   The Government Analyst under the Drugs and Cosmetics Act, 1940 (23 of 1940), of each participating State, ex officio, or where there is more than one in any such State, such one as the State Government may appoint in this behalf.

2. The agreement may provide that within the limits specified in clauses (a) and (b) of sub-section (1), the number of members to be elected or nominated under those clauses may or may not be the same in respect of each participating State.

3. Of the members, nominated by each State Government under clause (b) of sub-section (1), more than half shall be persons possessing a prescribed degree or diploma in pharmacy or pharmaceutical chemistry or registered pharmacists.

Incorporation of State Councils

Every State Council shall be a body corporate by such name as may be notified by the State Government in the Official Gazette or, in the case of a Joint State Council, as may be determined in the agreement, having perpetual succession and a common seal, with power to acquire or hold property both movable and immovable and shall by the said name sue and be sued.

President and Vice-President of State Council

1.   The President and Vice-President of the State Council be elected by the members from amongst themselves.

Provided that for five years from the first constitution of the State Council the President shall be a person nominated by the State Government who shall hold office at the pleasure of the State Government and where he is not already a member, shall be a member of the State Council in addition to the members referred to in section 19 or section 21, as the case may be.

2.   The President or Vice-President shall hold office as such for a term not exceeding five years and not extending beyond the expiry of his term as a member of the State Council, but subject to his being a member of the State Council, he shall be eligible for re-election.

Provided that if his term of office as a member of the State Council expires before the expiry of the full term for which he is elected as President or Vice-President, he shall, if he is re-elected or re-nominated as a member of the State Council, continue to hold office for the full term for which he is elected as President or Vice-President.

The council may appoint a registrar who acts as a secretary and such other staff as necessary.

The council have an executive committee consisting of-

1. The president.

2. The vice-president.

3. Other members.

The nominated and elected members of the council hold office for 5 years. A member who is absent from three consecutive meetings is to be deemed to have vacated his seat.

2.5 FUNCTIONS OF STATE PHARMACY COUNCIL

1. Registration of pharmacists in the state.

2. Preparation and maintenance of register.

3. Fix the rate of remuneration and allowance to its officers/members.

4. Inspection.

5. Mode of election.

A. REGISTRATION OF PHARMACISTS

The pharmacy act, 1948 provides for the registration of pharmacists through-

1. First register

2. Subsequent register.

FIRST REGISTER

State pharmacy council constitutes from the first register's registered pharmacists. Previously there was no provision for the registration, so there was no state pharmacy council. There were no registered pharmacists, though unofficial and unqualified persons were following/exploiting/performing the profession.

Preparation of first register

1. For the purpose of preparing the first register, the State Government shall by notification in the Official Gazette constitute a Registration Tribunal consisting of three persons, and shall also appoint a Registrar who shall act as Secretary of the Registration Tribunal.

2. The State Government shall, by the same or a like notification, appoint a date on or before which applications for registration, which shall be accompanied by the prescribed fee, shall be made to the Registration Tribunal.

3. The Registration Tribunal shall examine every application received on or before the appointed date, and if it is satisfied that the applicant is qualified for registration under section 31, shall direct the entry of the name of the applicant on the register.

4. The first register so prepared shall thereafter be published in such manner as the State Government may direct, and any person aggrieved by a decision of the Registration Tribunal expressed or implied in the register as so published may, within sixty days from the date of such publication, appeal to an authority appointed by the State Government in this behalf by notification in the Official Gazette.

5. The Registrar shall amend the register in accordance with the decisions of the authority appointed under sub-section (4) and shall thereupon issue to every person whose name is entered in the register a certificate of registration in the prescribed form.

6. Upon the constitution of the State Council, the register shall be given into its custody, and the State Government may direct that

all or any specified part of the application fees for registration in the first register shall be paid to the credit of the State Council.

Requirements for first register

1. Applicant should be at least 18 years of age.

2. Applicant should reside or carry on the business or profession of pharmacy in the concerned state.

Qualifications for entry on first register

A person who has attained the age of eighteen years shall be entitled on payment of the prescribed fee to have his name entered in the first register if he resides, or carries on the business or profession of pharmacy, in the State and if he-

1. Holds a degree or diploma in pharmacy or pharmaceutical chemistry or a chemist and druggist diploma of an Indian University or a State Government, as the case may be, or a prescribed qualification granted by an authority outside India, or

2. Holds a degree of an Indian University other than a degree in pharmacy or pharmaceutical chemistry, and has been engaged in the compounding of drugs in a hospital or dispensary or other place in which drugs are regularly dispensed on prescriptions of medical practitioners for a total period of not less than three years, or

3. Has passed an examination recognised as adequate by the State Government for compounders or dispensers, or

4. Has been engaged in the compounding of drugs in a hospital or dispensary or other place in which drugs are regularly dispensed on prescriptions of medical practitioners for a total period of not less than five years prior to the date notified under sub-section (2) of section 30.

SUBSEQUENT REGISTER

From the registered pharmacist of first register the constitution of the state council takes place. The first register and application fees are then handed over to state council.

Procedure for subsequent registration

1. After the formation of the state council applications are invited within a fixed (due) date, addressed to the registrar of the state council.

2. Upon receipt of the application, if the registrar is of the opinion that the applicant has the requisite qualification, he may direct his/her name to be entered in the register.

3. If any application has been rejected by registrar, he/she may appeal to the state council within 3 months of the rejection.

4. The decision of state council may be final.

Qualifications for subsequent registration

1. After the date appointed under sub-section (2) of section 30 and before the Education Regulations have, by or under section 11, taken effect in the State, a person who has attained the age of eighteen years shall on payment of the prescribed fee be entitled to have his name entered in the register if he resides or carries on the business or profession of pharmacy in the State and if he-

a. Satisfies the conditions prescribed with the prior approval of the Central Council, or where no conditions have been prescribed, the conditions entitling a person to have his name entered on the first register as set out in section 31, or

b. Is a registered pharmacist in another State, or

c. Possesses a qualification approved under section 14.

    Provided that no person shall be entitled under clause (a) of clause (c) to have his name entered on the register unless he has passed a matriculation examination or an examination prescribed as being equivalent to a matriculation examination.

2. After the Education Regulations have by or under section 11 taken effect in the State, a person shall on payment of the prescribed fee be entitled to have his name entered on the register if he has attained the age of eighteen years, if he resides, or

carries on the business or profession of pharmacy, in the State and if he has passed an approved examination or possesses a qualification approved under section 14 or is a registered pharmacist in another State.

SPECIAL PROVISIONS FOR REGISTRATION OF CERTAIN PERSONS

1. State Council may also permit to be entered on the register-

    a)   The names of displaced persons who have been carrying on the business or profession of pharmacy as their principal means of livelihood from a date prior to the 4th day of March, 1948, and who satisfy the conditions for registration as set out in section 31.

    b)   The names of citizens of India who have been carrying on the business or profession of pharmacy in any country outside India and who satisfy the conditions for registrations as set out in section 31.

    c)   The names of persons who resided in an area which has subsequently become a territory of India and who satisfy the conditions for registration as set out in section 31.

    d)   The names of persons who carry on the business or profession of pharmacy in the State, and

    > i. Would have satisfied the conditions for registration as set out in section 31, on the date appointed under sub-section (2) of section 30, had they applied for registration on or before that date; or

    > ii. Have been engaged in the compounding of drugs in a hospital or dispensary or other place in which drugs are regularly dispensed on prescriptions of medical practitioners as defined in sub-clause

    > iii. Of clause (f) of section 2 for a total period of not less than five years prior to the date appointed under sub-section (2) of section 30.

e)   The names of persons who were qualified to be entered in the register for a State as it existed immediately before the 1st day of November, 1956, but who, by reason of the area in which they resided or carried on their business or profession of pharmacy having become part of a State as formed on that date, are not qualified to be entered having in the register for the latter State only by reason of their not having passed either a matriculation examination or an examination prescribed as being equivalent to a matriculation examination or an approved examination or of their not possessing a qualification approved under section 14.

f)   The names of persons

i. Who were included in the register for a State as it existed immediately before the 1st day of November, 1956; and

ii. Who, by reason of the area in which they resided or carried on their business or profession of pharmacy having become part of a State as formed on that date, reside or carry on such business or profession in the latter State.

g)   The names of persons who reside or carry on their business of profession or pharmacy in an area in which this Chapter takes effect after the commencement of the Pharmacy (Amendment) Act, 1959, and who satisfy the conditions for registration as set out in section 31.

2. Any person who desires his name to be entered in the register in pursuance of sub-section (1) shall make an application in that behalf to the State Council, and such application shall be accompanied by the prescribed fee.

3. The provisions of this section shall remain in operation for a period of two years from the commencement of the Pharmacy (Amendment) Act, 1959.

Provided that the State Government may, by notification in the Official Gazette, extend the period of operation of clause (a), clause (b) or clause (c) of sub-section (1) by such further period or periods, not exceeding two years in the aggregate, as may be specified in the notification.

SPECIAL PROVISIONS FOR REGISTRATION OF DISPLACED PERSONS, REPATRIATES AND OTHER PERSONS

1. Notwithstanding anything contained in section 32 or section 32A, a State Council may permit to be entered on the register-

   a. The names of persons who possess the qualifications specified in clause (a) or clause (c) of section 31 and who were eligible for registration between the closing of the First Register and the date when the Education Regulations came into effect.

   b. the names of persons approved as "qualified persons" before the 31st December, 1969 for compounding or dispensing of medicines under the Drugs and Cosmetics Act, 1940 and the rules made thereunder.

   c. the names of displaced person or repatriates who were carrying on business or profession of pharmacy as their principal means of livelihood in any country outside India for a total period of not less than five years from a date prior to the date of application for registration.

2. The provisions of clauses (a) and (b) of sub–section (1) shall remain in operation for a period of two years from the commencement of the Pharmacy (Amendment) Act, 1976.

SCRUTINY OF APPLICATIONS FOR REGISTRATION

1. After the date appointed under sub-section (2) of section 30, applications for registration shall be addressed to the Registrar of the State Council and shall be accompanied by the prescribed fee.

2. If upon such application the Registrar is of opinion that the applicant is entitled to have his name entered in the register under

the provisions of this Act for the time being applicable, he shall enter the name of the applicant in the register:

Provided that no person whose name has under the provisions of this Act been removed from the register of any State shall be entitled to have his name entered in the register except with the approval of the State Council recorded at a meeting.

3. Any persons, whose application for registration is rejected by the Registrar, may within three months from the date of such rejection appeal to the State Council, and the decision of the State Council thereon shall be final.

4. Upon entry in the register of a name under section, the Registrar shall issue a certificate of registration in the prescribed form.

RENEWAL FEES

1. The State Government may, by notification in the Official Gazette, direct that for the retention of a name on the register after the 31st day of December of the year following the year in which the name is first entered on the register, there shall be paid annually to the State Council such renewal fee as may be prescribed, and where such direction has been made, such renewal fee shall be due to be paid before the first day of April of the year to which it relates.

2. Where a renewal fee is not paid by the due date, the Registrar shall remove the name of the defaulter from the register:

Provided that a name so removed may be restored to the register on such conditions as may be prescribed.

3. On payment of the renewal fee, the Registrar shall issue a receipt therefor and such receipt shall be proof of renewal of registration.

ENTRY OF ADDITIONAL QUALIFICATIONS

A registered pharmacist shall on payment of the prescribed fee be entitled to have entered in the register any further degrees or diplomas in pharmacy on pharmaceutical chemistry which he may obtain.

REMOVAL FROM REGISTER

1. Subject to the provisions of this section, the Executive Committee may order that the name of a registered pharmacist shall be removed from the register, where it is satisfied, after giving him a reasonable opportunity of being heard and after such further inquiry, if any, as it may think fit to make-

    i. that his name has been entered into the register by error or on account of misrepresentation or suppression of a material fact, or

    ii. that he has been convicted of any offence or has been guilty of any infamous conduct in any professional respect which in the opinion of the Executive Committee, renders him unfit to be kept in the register, or

    iii. that a person employed by him for the purposes of his business of pharmacy or employed to work under him in connection with any business of pharmacy has been convicted of any such offence or has been guilty of any such infamous conduct as would, if such person were a registered pharmacist, render him liable to have his name removed from the register under clause (ii).

    Provided that no such order shall be made under clause (iii) unless the Executive Committee is satisfied-

    a. that the offence or infamous conduct was instigated or connived at by the registered pharmacist, or

    b. that the registered pharmacist has at any time during the period or twelve months immediately preceding the date on which the offence or infamous conduct took place committed a similar offence or been guilty of similar infamous conduct, or

    c. that any person employed by the registered pharmacist for the purposes of his business of pharmacy or employed to work under him in connection with any business of pharmacy has at any time during the period of twelve months immediately preceding the date on which the offence or infamous conduct took place, committed a similar offence or been guilty of similar infamous conduct, and that the registered pharmacist had, or reasonably ought to have had, knowledge of such previous offence or infamous conduct , or

d. that where the offence or infamous conduct continued over a period, the registered pharmacist had, or reasonably ought to have had, knowledge of the continuing offence or infamous conduct, or

e. That where the offence is an offence under the Drugs and Cosmetics Act, 1940 , the registered pharmacist has not used due diligence in enforcing compliance with the provisions of that Act in his place of business and by persons employed by him or by persons under his control.

2. An order under sub-section (1) may direct that the person whose name is ordered to be removed from the register shall be ineligible for registration in the State under this Act either permanently or for such period as may be specified.

3. An order under sub-section (1) shall be subject to confirmation by the State Council and shall not take effect until the expiry of three month from the date of such confirmation.

4. A person aggrieved by an order under sub-section (1) which has been confirmed by the State Council may, within thirty days from the communication to him of such confirmation, appeal to the State Government, and the order of the State Government upon such appeal shall be final.

5. A person whose name has been removed from the register under this section or under sub-section (2) of section 34 shall forthwith surrender his certificate or registration to the Registrar, and the name so removed shall be published in the Official Gazette.

RESTORATION TO REGISTER

The State Council may at any time for reasons appearing to it sufficient order that upon payment of the prescribed fee the name of a person removed from the register shall be restored thereto:

Provided that where an appeal against such removal has been rejected by the State Government, an order under this section shall not take effect until it has been confirmed by the State Government.

BAR OF OTHER JURISDICTION

No order refusing to enter a name on the register or removing a name from the register shall be called in question in any Court.

ISSUE OF DUPLICATE CERTIFICATE OF REGISTRATION

Where it is shown to the satisfaction of the Registrar that a certificate of registration has been lost or destroyed, the Registrar may, on payment of the prescribed fee, issue a duplicate certificate in the prescribed form.

A.   PRINTING OF REGISTER AND EVIDENTIARY VALUE OF ENTRIES THEREIN

1. As soon as may be after the 1st day of April subsequent to the commencement of the Pharmacy (Amendment) Act, 1959 (24 of 1959), the Registrar shall cause to be printed copies of the register as it stood on the said date.

2. The Registrar shall thereafter cause to be printed as soon as may be after the 1st day of April in each year copies of the annual supplement to the register referred to in sub-section (1), showing all additions to and other amendments in, the said register.

3. Then,

   a)   The register shall be brought up-to-date three months before ordinary elections to the State Council are held and copies of this register shall be printed.

   b)   The provisions of sub-section (2) shall apply to the register as so printed as they apply to the register referred to in sub-section (1).

4. The copies referred to in sub-section (1) or sub-section (2) or sub-section (3) shall be made be available to persons applying therefor on payment of the prescribed charge and shall be evidence that on the date referred to in the register or annual

supplement, as the case may be, the persons whose name are entered therein were registered pharmacists.

B.   PREPARATION AND MAINTENANCE OF REGISTER

1. As soon as may be after this chapter has taken effect in any State, the State Government shall cause to be prepared in the manner hereinafter provided a register of pharmacists for the State.

2. The State Council shall as soon as possible after it is constituted assume the duty of maintaining the register in accordance with the provisions of this Act.

3. The register shall include the following particulars, namely-

    a. The full name and residential address of the registered person.

    b. The date of his first admission to the register.

    c. His qualifications for registration.

    d. His professional address, and if he is employed by any person, the name of such person.

    e. Such further particulars as may be prescribed.

C.   STAFF, REMUNERATION AND ALLOWANCES

The State Council may, with the previous sanction of the State Government,-

1. Appoint a Registrar who shall also act as Secretary and, if so decided by the State Council, Treasurer, of the State Council.

2. Appoint such other officers and servants as may be required to enable the State Council to carry out its functions under this Act.

3. Fix the salaries and allowances and other conditions of service of the Secretary and other officers and servants of the State Council.

4. Fix the rates of allowances payable to members of the State Council.

Provided that for the first four years from the first constitution of the State Council, the Registrar shall be a person appointed by the State Government, who shall hold office during the pleasure of the State Government.

D.   INSPECTION

1. A State Council may, with the previous sanction of the State Government, appoint Inspectors having the prescribed qualifications.

2. An Inspector may-

   a. Inspect any premises where drugs are compounded or dispensed and submit a written report to the Registrar.

   b. Enquire whether a person who is engaged in compounding or dispensing of drugs is a registered pharmacist.

   c. Investigate any complaint made in writing in respect of any contravention of this Act and report to the Registrar.

   d. Institute prosecution under the order of the Executive Committee of the State Council.

   e. Exercise such other powers as may be necessary for carrying out the purposes of this Act or any rules made thereunder.

3. Any person wilfully obstructing an Inspector in the exercise of the powers conferred on him by or under this Act or any rules made thereunder shall be punishable with imprisonment for a term which may extend to six months, or with fine not exceeding one thousand rupees, or with both.

4. Every Inspector shall be deemed to be a public servant within the meaning of section 21 of the Indian Penal Code (45 of 1860).

E.   MODE OF ELECTIONS

Elections under this Chapter shall be conducted in the prescribed manner, and where any dispute arises regarding any such election, it shall be referred to the State Government whose decision shall be final.

S.No	OFFENCES	PENALTIES
1.	False claiming to be a registered pharmacist.	A Fine upto Rs 500/- on first conviction. B Fine of Rs 1000/- and/or 6 months imprisonment of any subsequent conviction.
2.	Dispended by unregistered pharmacists.	6 months imprisonment or Rs 1000/- fine or both
3.	Failure to surrender Certificate of Registration.	Fine upto Rs 50/-
4.	Obstructing State pharmacy council inspectors.	6 months imprisonment or Rs 1000/- fine or both.

REVIEW QUESTIONS

ESSAY QUESTIONS

1. Explain the Constitution and Functions of Pharmacy council of India.

2. Write the Constitution and Function of Provisional Pharmacy council of India.

SHORT QUESTIONS

1. Define the following.
a) Registered medical practitioner.
b) Registered pharmacist.
2. Write a note on Registration of Pharmacists through First register.
3. Write a note on Registration of Pharmacists through subsequent register.

4.   Write a note on Scrutiny of applications for registration and Renewal fees.

5.   Write a note on Removal of name from the Register.

6.   Enumerate various Offences and Penalties under the Pharmacy Act 1948.

MCQ's

1.   In which year was the pharmacy act passed?
   a) 1947
   b) 1948
   c) 1974
   d) 1984

2.   P.C.I
   a) Pharmacy committee of India.
   b) Pharmacy council of India.
   c) Central council of India.
   d) Both b and c

3.   Director General of Health Service is,
   a) Ex-officio member.
   b) Elected member.
   c) Nominated member.
   d) President of executive committee.

4.   The executive committee of P.C.I consist of how many members?
   a) 3
   b) 5
   c) 7
   d) 8

5.   Which of the following is the function of P.C.I?
   a) Education regulation.
   b) Application of Education Regulations to States.

c) Preparation of Central Register.

d) All of the above.

6. How many elected members are present in Separate State Council?

a) 3

b) 5

c) 7

d) 9

7. Chief Administrative Medical Officer of the State Pharmacy Council is

a) Elected members.

b) Nominated members.

c) Ex-officio members.

d) None of these.

8. What is the age of the applicant requirement in order to enter the State Register?

a) 21

b) 20

c) 19

d) 18

9. The treasurer of the state council is

a) President.

b) Vice-president.

c) Registrar.

d) Any of the Ex-officio members.

10. The registration tribunal constituted state government for preparation of first register consists of

a) 2 members.

b) 3 members.

c) 5 members.

d) 7 members.

Chapter 3

DRUGS AND COSMETICS ACT, 1940 AND RULES, 1945

3.1 INTRODUCTION

1. This Act may be called the Drugs and Cosmetics Act, 1940.

2. It extends to the whole of India.

3. It shall come into force at once; but shall take the effect only from such a date as the Central Government may, by notification in the Official Gazette, appoint in this behalf, and those related to Ayurvedic, Siddha and Unani drugs shall take effect in a particular State only from such a date as the State Government may, by like notification, appoint in this behalf.

4. Originally the Drugs and Cosmetics Act was passed in 1940. Then subsequently amended as follows,

   a) The Repealing and Amending Act, 1949.

   b) The Adaptation of laws order, 1950.

   c) The Drugs (Amendment) Act, 1960.

   d) The Drugs (Amendment) Act, 1962.

   e) The Drugs (Amendment) Act, 1964.

   f) The Drugs and Cosmetics (Amendment) Act, 1972.

   g) The Drugs and Cosmetics (Amendment) Act, 1982.

   h) The Drugs and Cosmetics (Amendment) Act, 1995.

   i) The Drugs and Cosmetics (Amendment) Act, 1999.

OBJECTIVES

1.   To regulate the Import, Manufacture, Distribution and Sale of Drugs and Cosmetics.

2.   Provide licenee for Manufacture and Sale of Drugs and Cosmetics.

3.   To prevent substandard in drugs, presumably for maintaining high standard of Medical treatment.

4.   To regulate the Manufacture and Sale of Ayurvedic, Siddha and Unani drugs.

5.   Establishment of Drugs Technical Advisory Board and Ayurvedic, Siddha and Unani Drugs Technical Advisory Board and Drugs Consultative Committees for Allopathic and Ayurvedic.

DEFINITIONS

1.   *Ayurvedic, Siddha or Unani drugs:* Includes all medicines intended for internal or external use for or in the diagnosis, treatment, mitigation or prevention of disease or disorder in human beings or animals, and manufactured exclusively in accordance with the formulae described in, the authoritative books of Ayurvedic, Siddha and Unani (Tibb) systems of medicine, specified in the First Schedule.

2.   *Cosmetic:* Means any article intended to be rubbed, poured, sprinkled or sprayed on, or introduced into, or otherwise applied to, the human body or any part thereof for cleansing, beautifying, promoting attractiveness, or altering the appearance, and includes any article intended for use as a component of cosmetic.

3.   *Drug:* Includes

a)   All medicines for internal or external use of human beings or animals and all substances intended to be used for or in the diagnosis, treatment, mitigation or prevention of any disease or disorder in human beings or animals, including preparations applied on human body for the purpose of repelling insects like mosquitoes;

b)   Such substances (other than food) intended to affect the structure or any function of human body or intended to be used for the destruction of vermin or insects which cause disease in human beings or animals, as may be specified from time to time by the Central Government by notification in the Official Gazette;

c) All substances intended for use as components of a drug including empty gelatine capsules; and

d) Such devices intended for internal or external use in the diagnosis, treatment, mitigation or prevention of disease or disorder in human beings or animals, as may be specified from time to time by the Central Government by notification in the Official Gazette, after consultation with the Board.

6. *Adulterated drugs:* Means drugs containing filthy, putrid or decomposed substances or colours other than those prescribed or drugs processed and stored under conditions which are likely to make them injurious to health or drugs packed in containers composed of poisonous or deleterious substances of drugs which contain any harmful or toxic substances which make them injurious to health or drugs which have been mixed up with any substance likely to reduce their quality or strength.

7. *Misbranded drugs:* Drugs coloured, coated, powdered or polished so as to conceal damage or to make it appear of better quality value than they really are or drugs which are false or misleading in claims or drugs not labelled in the prescribed manner or imported in name of other drug.

8. *New drugs:* Drugs whose composition is generally not recognised as safe for use under the conditions recommended or suggested in the label and drugs whose composition is recognised as safe but which have not been used to any large extent or appreciable period of time.

9. *Spurious drugs:* Drugs which are imported under the name of other drug or drugs which are imitation or substituent for other drugs or resemble other drugs in a manner likely to cause cheating or bear names of manufacturers which are made-up fictitious and of whom they are truly not the product or drugs which have been partly or wholly substituted by other substances or drugs.

10. **Standard drugs:** Means drugs complying with standards prescribed in the drug and cosmetic Act.

11. **Drug store:** Premises licensed for the sale of drugs which need not have a qualified person.

12. **Government Analyst:** Means—

a)   In relation to Ayurvedic, Siddha or Unani drug, a Government Analyst appointed by Central Government or a State Government under section 33F; and

b)   In relation to any other drug or cosmetic, a Government Analyst appointed by the Central Government or a State Government under section.

13. **Inspector:** Means

a.   In relation to Ayurvedic, Siddha or Unani drug, an Inspector appointed by the Central Government or a State Government under section 33G; and

b.   In relation to any other drug or cosmetic, an Inspector appointed by the Central Government or a State Government under section 2.

14. **Manufacture:** In relation to any drug or cosmetic includes any process or part of a process for making, altering, ornamenting, finishing, packing, labelling, breaking up or otherwise treating or adopting any drug or cosmetic with a view to its sale or distribution but does not include the compounding or dispensing of any drug, or the packing of any drug or cosmetic, in the ordinary course of retail business; and "to manufacture" shall be construed accordingly.

15. **To import:** Means to bring into India.

16. **Patent or proprietary medicine:** means,

a)   In relation to Ayurvedic, Siddha or Unani Tibb systems of medicine   all formulations containing only such ingredients mentioned in the formulae described in the authoritative books of Ayurveda, Siddha or Unani Tibb systems of medicine specified in the First Schedule, but does not include a medicine which is administered by parentral route and also a formulation included in the authoritative books as specified in clause *(a)*;

b) In relation to any other systems of medicine, a drug which is a remedy or prescription presented in a form ready for internal or external administration of human beings or animals and which is not included in the edition of Indian Pharmacopoeia for the time being or any other Pharmacopoeia authorized in this behalf by Central Government after consultation with the Drugs Technical Advisory Board constituted under section 5.

17. *Export:* Means to take out of India across any of the custom frontiers (ports).

18. *Pharmacy:* Premises licensed for the retail sale of drugs which have the qualified person and engaged in compounding of drugs by maintaining pharmacy.

19. *Qualified person:* person holding degree or diploma in pharmacy or pharmaceutical chemistry or registered as pharmacist under the pharmacy act or having not less than four years experience of dispensing or a qualified person before 31/12/1969.

20. *Repacking of drugs:* Process of breaking up of any drug from a bulk container into small packages and labelling of these packages with a view to their sale and distribution.

21. *Spurious cosmetics:* Means,

a) Cosmetics which are imitation or substituent for another cosmetic or resemble another cosmetic in a manner likely to cause cheating or upon its label or container the name of another cosmetic.

b) If it is imported under name of another cosmetics or bear names of manufacturers who are truly not their manufacturers.

c) If the label or container bears the name of an individual or a company purporting to be the manufacturer of the cosmetic which individual or company is fictitious or does not exist.

d) If it purports to be the product of a manufacturer of whom it is not truly a product.

22. **Misbranded cosmetics:** Any cosmetics is said to be misbranded,

a) If it contains a colour which is not prescribed.

b) If it is not labelled in prescribed manner.

c) If the label or container or anything accompanying the cosmetics bear statement which is false or misleading in any particular.

23. **Loan licence:** It means a licence issued by a licensing authority to person who does not have his own arrangement for manufacture but who intends to avail himself of the manufacturing facilities owned by another manufacturer.

24. **Standard quality:** In relation to drug it means that the drug complies with the standard set out in the second schedule, and in relation to cosmetics, that the cosmetic complies with such standards as may be prescribed.

3.2 ADMINISRATION OF THE ACT

ADVISORY

A. **The Drugs Technical Advisory Board (DTAB):**

1. The Central Government shall, as soon as may be, constitute a Board (to be called the Drugs Technical Advisory Board) to advise the Central Government and the State Governments on technical matters arising out of the administration of this Act and to carry out the other functions assigned to it by this Act.

The Board shall consist of the following members, namely,

a) The Director General of Health Services, ex officio, who shall be Chairman;

b) The Drugs Controller, India ex officio ;

c) The Director of the Central Drugs Laboratory, Calcutta, ex-officio;

d) The Director of the Central Research Institute, Kasauli, ex-officio;

e)   The Director of the Indian Veterinary Research Institute, Izatnagar, ex-officio ;

f)   The President of the Medical Council of India, ex-officio;

g)   The President of the Pharmacy Council of India, ex-officio ;

h)   The Director of the Central Drug Research Institute, Lucknow, ex-officio;

i)   Two persons to be nominated by the Central Government from among persons who are in charge of drugs control in the States ;

j)   One person, to be elected by the Executive Committee of the Pharmacy Council of India, from among teachers in pharmacy or pharmaceutical chemistry or pharmacognosy on the staff of an Indian university or a college affiliated thereto;

k)   One person, to be elected by the Executive Committee of the Medical Council of India, from among teachers in medicine or therapeutics on the staff of an Indian university or a college affiliated thereto ;

l)   One person to be nominated by the Central Government from the pharmaceutical industry ;

m)   One pharmacologist to be elected by the Governing Body of the Indian Council of Medical Research ;

n)   One person to be elected by the Central Council of the Indian Medical Association ;

o)   One person to be elected by the Council of the Indian Pharmaceutical Association ;

p)   Two persons holding the appointment of Government Analyst under this Act, to be nominated by the Central Government.

2.   The nominated and elected members of the Board shall hold office for three years, but shall be eligible for re-nomination and re-election

3.   The Board may, subject to the previous approval of the Central Government, make bye-laws fixing a quorum and regulating its own procedure and the conduct of all business to be transacted by it.

4. The Board may constitute sub-committees and may appoint to such sub-committees for such periods, not exceeding three years, as it may decide, or temporarily for the consideration of particular matters, persons who are not members of the Board.

5. The functions of the Board may be exercised notwithstanding any vacancy therein.

6. The Central Government shall appoint a person to be Secretary of the Board and shall provide the Board with such clerical and other staff as the Central Government considers necessary.

Functions:

1. To advise the Central Government and State Government on technical matters.

2. Modification and Amendments in the Act with consultation of board.

3. Any other functions assigned.

B. ***The Drugs Consultative Committee:***

1. The Central Government may constitute an advisory committee to be called "the Drugs Consultative Committee" to advise the Central Government, the State Governments and the Drugs Technical Advisory Board on any matter tending to secure uniformity throughout India in the administration of this Act.

2. The Drugs Consultative Committee shall consist of two representatives of the Central Government to be nominated by that Government and one representative of each State Government to be nominated by the State Government concerned.

3. The Drugs Consultative Committee shall meet when required to do so by the Central Government and shall have power to regulate its own procedure.

Functions:

1. To secure uniformity in the act throughout India.

2. To advise the various Government and DTAB.

ANALYTICAL

A. *The Central Drugs Laboratory (CDL):*

1. The Central Government shall, as soon as may be, establish a Central Drugs Laboratory under the control of a Director to be appointed by the Central Government, to carry out the functions entrusted to it by this Act or any rules made under this Chapter :

   Provided that, if the Central government so prescribes, the functions of the Central Drugs Laboratory in respect of any drug or class of drugs or cosmetic or class of cosmetics] or class of cosmetics shall be carried out at the Central Research Institute, Kasauli, or at any other prescribed Laboratory and the functions of the Director of the Central Drugs Laboratory in respect of such drug or class of or such cosmetic or class of cosmetics shall be exercised by the Director of that Institute or of that other Laboratory, as the case may be.

2. The Central Government may, after consultation with the Board, make rules prescribing –

   a) The functions of the Central Drugs Laboratory ;

   b) The procedure for the submission of the said Laboratory of samples of drugs or cosmetics for analysis or test, the forms of the Laboratory's reports thereon and the fees payable in respect of such reports ;

   c) Such other matters as may be necessary or expedient to enable the said Laboratory to carry out its functions ;

   d) The matters necessary to be prescribed for the purposes of the proviso to sub-section (1).

B. *Government analyst:*

1. The State Government may, by notification in the Official Gazette, appoint such persons as it thinks fit, having the prescribed qualifications, to be Government Analysts for such areas in the

state and in respect of such drugs or classes of drug or such cosmetics or classes of cosmetics as may specified in the notification.

2.   The Central Government may also, by notification in the Official Gazette, appoint such persons as it thinks fit, having the prescribed qualifications, to be Government Analysts in respect of such drugs or classes of drugs or such cosmetics or classes of cosmetics as may be specified in the notification.

3.   Notwithstanding anything contained in sub-section (*1*) or sub-section (*2*), neither the Central Government nor a State Government shall appoint as a Government Analyst any official not serving under it without the previous consent of the Government under which he is serving.

4.   No person who has any financial interest in the import, manufacture or sale of drugs or cosmetics shall be appointed to be a Government Analyst under sub-section *(1)* or subsection *(2)* of this section.

Qualification:

1.   For Analysis/Testing of other than Biological (C/C$_1$):

•   A Graduate in Medicine or Science or Pharmacy or Pharmaceutical chemistry and with at least 5 years of post graduate experience in testing; or

•   A Post Graduate degree in Medicine or Science or Pharmacy or Pharmaceutical chemistry and with at least 3 years of experience in testing; or

•   Holding Associate ship Diploma of the institution of chemists with Analysis of drugs and Pharmaceuticals and with at least 3 years of experience in testing.

2.   For analysis/testing of biological (C/C$_1$):

•   A Graduate in Medicine or Science or Pharmacy or Pharmaceutical chemistry and trained either in physiology, bacteriology, serology, pathology, pharmacology, or microbiology and with at least 5 years of post graduate experience in testing of biological products; or

- A Post Graduate degree in Medicine or Science or Pharmacy or Pharmaceutical chemistry or Associate ship diploma of the institution of chemists with Analysis of drugs and Pharmaceuticals and trained either in physiology, bacteriology, serology, pathology, pharmacology, or microbiology and with at least 3 years of experience in testing of biological.

3. For analysis/testing of biological for veterinary use:

- A Graduate in Veterinary Science or General Science or Medicine or Pharmacy and with at least 5 years experience of testing.

- A Post Graduate in Veterinary Science or General Science or Medicine or Pharmacy or Pharmaceutical Chemistry and with at least 3 years experience of testing.

Duties:

1. To analyze and test samples of drugs and cosmetics sent by drug inspector or other persons and furnish the reports.

2. To engage in any research work and forward the report to the government with a view to publication.

Procedure:

1. On receipt of samples the analyst should record the condition or the seal and compare it with the impression of the seal received separately.

2. After completion of the analysis, a report in triplicate with full details should be supplied.

EXECUTIVE

A. *Licensing authority:*

1. For import of drugs and cosmetics, the central government appoints licensing authorities to issue licences.

2. For manufacture and sale of drugs and cosmetics, the state government appoints licensing authority for respective territories to issue licences.

3.   The licensing authority are designated differently in different states as follows,

- Drug controller.

- Director.

- Drug control administrator.

- Officer in charge, drug control.

- Commissioner- FDCA.

Qualifications:

A graduate in Pharmacy or Pharmaceutical chemistry or Medicine (clinical pharmacology) or Microbiology and with at least 5 years of experience in manufacture or testing of drug or enforcement of the Act.

B.   Controlling authorities:

All inspectors appointed shall be under the control of a controlling authority.

Qualifications:

A graduate in Pharmacy or Pharmaceutical chemistry or Medicine (clinical pharmacology) or Microbiology and with at least 5 years of experience in manufacture or testing of drug or enforcement of the Act.

C.   Drug inspectors:

1. The Central Government or a State Government may, by notification in the Official Gazette, appoint such person as it thinks fit, having the prescribed qualification, to be Inspectors for such areas as may be assigned to them by the Central Government or State Government, as the case may be.

2. The powers which may be exercised by an Inspector and the duties which may be performed by him, the drugs or classes of drugs or cosmetics or classes of cosmetics in relation to which and the conditions, limitations or restrictions subject to which, such powers and duties may be exercised or performed shall be such as may be prescribed.

3. No person who has any financial interest in the import, manufacture or sale of drugs or cosmetics shall be appointed to be an Inspector under this section.

4. Every Inspector shall be deemed to be public servant within the meaning of section 21 of the Indian Penal Code (45 of 1860), and shall be officially subordinate to such authority having the prescribed qualification as the Government appointing him may specify in this behalf.

Qualifications:

1. To inspect premises manufacturing biological and other than biological:

   a. A degree in Pharmacy or Pharmaceutical chemistry or

   b. Pharm. Science; or

   c. Diploma of the Institution of chemist (India); or

   d. Degree in Medicine, Clinical pharmacology or Microbiology.

With the above qualifications and,

   a. Not less than 18 months experience in the manufacturing or testing of the substances specified in schedule C; or

   b. Not less than 3 years experience in the inspection of firm manufacturing any of the substances specified in schedule C.

2. To inspect premises manufacturing biological (Veterinary):

   a. A Graduate in Veterinary science or Medicine or General science or Pharmacy and 18 months experience in the manufacturing or testing of Veterinary biological; or

   b. A Graduate in Veterinary science or Medicine or General science or Pharmacy and 3 years experience in the inspection of firm manufacturing Veterinary biological.

Powers of Inspectors:

1. Subject to the provisions of section 23 and of any rules made by the Central Government in this behalf, an Inspector may, within the local limits of the area for which he is appointed,

    a) For clauses (a), (b) and (c) inspect,

        •   Any premises wherein any drug or cosmetic is being manufactured and the means employed for stand arising and testing the drug or cosmetic;

        •   Any premises wherein any drug or cosmetic is being sold, or stocked or exhibited or offered for sale, or distributed;

    b) Take samples of any drug or cosmetic, -

        •   Which is being manufactured or being sold or is stocked or exhibited or offered for sale, or is being distributed;

        •   From any person who is in the course of conveying, delivering or preparing to deliver such drug or cosmetic to a purchaser or a consignee;

    c) At all reasonable times, with such assistance, if any, as he considers necessary, -

        •   Search any person, who, he has reason to believe, has secreted about his person, any drug or cosmetic in respect of which an offence under this Chapter has been, or is being, committed; or

        •   Enter and search any place in which he has reason to believe that an offence under this Chapter has been, or is being, committed; or

        •   Stop and search any vehicle, vessel or other conveyance which, he has reason to believe, is being used for carrying any drug or cosmetic in respect of which an offence under this Chapter has been, or is being, committed, and order in writing the person in possession of the drug or cosmetic in respect of which the offence has been, or is being, committed, not to dispose of any stock of such drug or cosmetic for a specified period not exceeding twenty days, or, unless the alleged offence is such that the defect may be removed by the possessor of the drug or cosmetic, seize the stock of such drug or cosmetic and any substance or article by means of which the offence has been, or is being committed or which may be employed for the commission of such offence;

Examine any record, register, document or any other material object found for certain words with any person, or in any place, vehicle, vessel or other conveyance referred to in clause (c), and seize the same if he has reason to believe that it may furnish evidence of the commission of an offence punishable under this Act or the rules made thereunder;

Require any person to produce any record, register, or other document relating to the manufacture for sale or for distribution, stocking, exhibition for sale, offer for sale or distribution of any drug or cosmetic in respect of which he has reason to believe that an offence under this Chapter has been, or is being, or is being, committed;

d)   Exercise such other powers as may be necessary for carrying out the purposes of this Chapter or any rules made there under.

2.   The provisions of the Code of Criminal Procedure, 1973 shall, so far as may be, apply to any search or seizure under this Chapter as they apply to any search or seizure made under the authority of a warrant issued under section 94 of the said Code.

Every record, register or other document seized under clause (c) or produced under clause (c) shall be returned to the person, from whom they were seized or who produce the same, within a period of twenty days of the date of such seizure or production, as the case may be, after copies thereof or extracts therefrom certified by that person, in such manner as may be prescribed, have been taken.

3.   If any person wilfully obstructs an Inspector in the exercise of the powers conferred upon him by or under this Chapter refuses to produce any record, register or other document when so required under clause (c) of sub-section (1), he shall be punishable with

imprisonment which may extend to three years, or with fine, or with both.

Procedure of Inspectors:

1. Where an Inspector takes any sample of a drug or cosmetic under this Chapter, he shall tender the fair price thereof and may require a written acknowledgement therefore.

2. Where the price tendered under sub-section (1) is refused, or where the Inspector seizes the stock of any drug or cosmetic under clause (c) of section 22, he shall tender a receipt therefore in the prescribed form.

3. Where an Inspector takes a sample of a drug or cosmetic for the purpose of test or analysis, he shall intimate such purpose in writing in the prescribed form to the person from whom he takes it and, in the presence of such person unless he wilfully absents himself, shall divide the sample into four portions and effectively seal and suitably mark the same and permit such person to add his own seal and mark to all or any of the portions so sealed and marked.

    Provided that where the sample is taken from premises whereon the drug or cosmetic is being manufactured, it shall be necessary to divide the sample into three portions only.

    Provided further that where the drug or cosmetic is made up in containers of small volume, instead of dividing a sample as aforesaid, the Inspector may, and if the drug or cosmetic be such that it is likely to deteriorate or be otherwise damaged by exposure shall, take three or four, as the case may be, of the said containers after suitably marking the same and, where necessary sealing them.

4. The Inspector shall restore one portion of a sample so divided or one container, as the case may be, to the person from whom he takes it, and shall retain the remainder and dispose of the same as follows :-

    i.   One portion or container he shall forthwith send to the Government Analyst for test or analysis ;

ii.   The second he shall produce to the Court before which proceedings, if any, are instituted in respect of the drug or cosmetic; and

iii.   The third, where taken, he shall send to the person, if any, whose name, address and other particulars have been disclosed under section 18A.

5.   Where an Inspector takes any action under clause (c) of section 22,

a)   He shall use all dispatch in ascertaining whether or not the drug or cosmetic contravenes any of the provisions of section 18 and, if it is ascertained that the drug or cosmetic does not so contravene, forthwith revoke the order passed under the said clause or, as the case may be, taken such action as may be necessary for the return of the stock-seized ;

b)   If he seizes the stock of the drug or cosmetic, he shall as soon as may be inform a Judicial Magistrate and take his orders as to the custody thereof;

c)   Without prejudice to the institution of any prosecution, if the alleged contravention be such that the defect may be remedied by the possessor of the drug or cosmetic, he shall, on being satisfied that the defect has been so remedied, forthwith revoke his order under the said clause.

6.   Where an Inspector seizes any record, register, document or any other material object under clause (c) of sub-section (1) of section 22, he shall, as soon as may be, inform a Judicial Magistrate and take his orders as to the custody thereof.

3.3 SCHEDULES TO THE ACT

There are two schedules to the act.

a) **First schedule:** Names of books under Ayurvedic and Siddha systems.

b) **Second schedule:** Standards to be complied with, by imported drugs and by drugs manufactured for sale or distribution.

SCHEDULES TO THE RULES

There are several schedules to the rules as shown in the table below,

S.NO	TYPES	CONTENTS
1.	Schedule A	Applications for licenses for import, mfg., and sale of drug and cosmetics, the forms in which the licenses are granted and renewed and other forms.
2.	Schedule B	Fees for analysis of drug and cosmetics that have to be paid to the Central Drug Laboratories or other Government Laboratories.
3.	Schedule C	List of Biological and Immunological Products, Antibiotics and Ophthalmic lotions and Ointments and all products for parentral use (injections).
4.	Schedule C_1	List of drugs, from biological origin, namely Alkaloids, Hormones, Vitamins and Antibiotics for oral use.
5.	Schedule D	Exemptions that have been granted to drugs and importers of drugs from complying with the requirements of import of drugs and also the conditions for such exemptions.
6.	Schedule E	List of poisons for which labelling and other requirements were to be complied with. This schedule has been deleted.
7.	Schedule E_1	List of poisonous substances under the Ayurvedic, Siddha and Unani Systems of medicines.
8.	Schedule F (F_i, F_{ii})	Special provisions to be complied with, for the manufacture, testing and labelling of biological products for human use like Sera and Vaccines. These provisions have now been deleted. The requirements for running Blood Banks and other requirements are now includes in this schedule.

Continued on next page

S.NO	TYPES	CONTENTS
9.	Schedule F$_1$	Special provisions to be complied with for the manufacture, testing and labelling of Veterinary Biological Products.
10.	Schedule F$_2$	Standards for Surgical Dressings.
11.	Schedule F$_3$	Standards for Umbilical Tapes.
12.	Schedule FF	Additional standards for ophthalmic preparations.
13.	Schedule G	List of drugs which should be used by patient under medical supervision and which shall be labelled with the words "Caution – It is dangerous to take this preparation except under medical supervision".
14.	Schedule H	List of drugs which are to be sold by retail against the prescription of Registered Medical Practitioner and which shall be labelled with words "Schedule H Drug- Warning: to be sold by retail on the prescription of a Registered Medical Practitioner only."
15.	Schedule I	List of poisons of particulars about the proportion of poison in certain cases. Schedule I was linked with Schedule E. When schedule E was deleted in 1982, Schedule I was also deleted.
16.	Schedule J	Names of diseases and ailments (by whatever name described) which a drug may not purpose to prevent or cure by means of claims made on the label of the container of the drug.
17.	Schedule K	Names of drugs or classes of drugs which are exempted from complying with the provisions for manufacture, sale and standards of drugs and the conditions of such exemption.

Continued on next page

S.NO	TYPES	CONTENTS
18.	Schedule L	List of drugs which were required to be sold by retail against the prescription of Registered Medical Practitioner. Subsequently the drugs listed in Schedule L were transferred to Schedule H. Schedule L was deleted in 1982.
19.	Schedule M	**Good Manufacturing Practices (GMP) and the** **requirements of premises, plant and equipments for** **manufacture of drugs.**
20.	Schedule M$_1$	Requirements for factory premises of Homeopathic Medicines.
21.	Schedule M$_2$	Requirements for factory premises of Cosmetics.
22.	Schedule M$_3$	Requirements of factory premises for manufacture of Medical Devices.
23.	Schedule N	List of minimum equipments, requirements of premises for the effective running of a pharmacy.
24.	Schedule O	Standards for Disinfectant fluids.
25.	Schedule P	Life Period and Conditions of Storage of Drugs.
26.	Schedule P$_1$	Pack sizes of Drugs.
27.	Schedule Q	List of Coal Tar colours permitted to be used in cosmetics.
28.	Schedule Q$_1$	Use of permitted colours in soaps.
29.	Schedule R	Standards and labelling requirements of Condoms, Copper-T and Contraceptive Tube Rings.
30.	Schedule R$_1$	Standards to be complied with by medical devices.
31.	Schedule S	Standards for Cosmetics.
32.	Schedule T	Requirements of factory premises and hygienic conditions to be complied with by the manufacturer of Ayurvedic, Siddha and Unani Drugs.

Continued on next page

S.NO	TYPES	CONTENTS
33.	Schedule U	Particulars to be shown in the manufacturing records, record of raw materials and in the analytical records of drugs.
34.	Schedule U_1	Particulars to be shown in the manufacturing records, record of raw materials and in the analytical records of cosmetics.
35.	Schedule V	Standards for patient and proprietary medicines and the maximum and minimum quantities of vitamins that are permitted to be added in such preparations for oral use.
36.	Schedule W	Names of drugs which shall be marketed under generic names only.
37.	Schedule X	Names of psychotropic drugs for which special control measures have been laid down.
38.	Schedule Y	Requirements and guidelines on clinical trials for import and manufacture of new drugs.

3.4 IMPORT

PROHIBITION OF IMPORT OF CERTAIN DRUGS OR COSMETICS

From such date as may be fixed by the Central Government by notification in the Official Gazette in this behalf, no person shall import,

1. Any drug or cosmetic which is not of standard quality.

2. Any misbranded drug or misbranded (or spurious) cosmetic.

3. Any adulterated (or spurious) drug.

4. Any drug or cosmetic for the import of which a licence is prescribed, otherwise than under, and in accordance with, such licence.

5. Any patent or proprietary medicine, unless there is displayed in the prescribed manner on the label or container thereof the true formula or list of active ingredients contained in it, together with the quantities thereof.

6. Any drug which by means of any statement, design or device accompanying it or by any other means, purports or claims to cure or mitigate any such disease or ailment, or to have any such other effect, as may be prescribed.

7. Any cosmetic containing any ingredient which may render it unsafe or harmful for use under the directions indicated or recommended.

8. Any drug or cosmetic the import of which is prohibited by rule made under this Chapter.

Provided that nothing in this section shall apply to the import, subject to prescribed conditions, of small quantities of any drug for the purpose of examination, test or analysis or for personal use.

Provided further that the Central Government may, after consultation with the Board, by notification in the Official Gazette, permit, subject to any conditions specified in the notification, the import of any drug or class of drugs not being of standard quality.

IMPORT OF DRUGS UNDER LICENCE

1. Licence is required for the import of drugs.

2. Licence is obtained on application to the proper licensing authority (Custom Collector/ Drug Controller of India).

3. Licence is valid up to 31st December.

4. Licensee should inform to licensing authority, if any changes.

IMPORT OF BIOLOGICAL DRUGS (C/C_1)

Conditions to be fulfilled:

1. Licensee must have adequate facilities for storage.

2. Licensee must maintain a record of the sale, showing the particulars of the names of drugs and of the persons to whom they have been sold.

3. Licensee must allow an inspector to inspect premises and to check the records.

4. Licensee must furnish the sample to the authority.

5. Licensee must not sell the drugs from which sample is withdrawn and he is advised not to sale, or recall the batch from the market.

6. Licensee must comply with undertaking given in Form No: 09

7. Licensee must inform the licensing authority about any change in constitution of licensed firm.

IMPORT OF SCHEDULE-X DRUGS

Conditions to be fulfilled:

1. A license is necessary.

2. Licensee must have adequate facilities for storage.

3. Applicant must be reputable in the occupation, trade or business.

4. The license granted ever before should not be suspended or cancelled.

5. The licensee has not been convicted any offence under the Drugs and Cosmetic Act or Narcotic and Psychotropic Substances Act.

IMPORT OF DRUGS FOR EXAMINATION, TEST OR ANALYSIS

Condition to be fulfilled:

1. A licence is necessary.

2. Imported under licence in Form-11.

3. The licensee must use the imported drug only for the said purpose and use at the place specified in the licence.

4. The licensee must keep the record to the quantities, name of the manufacturer and date of import.

5. The licensee must allow an Inspector to inspect the premises and check the records.

DRUGS IMPORTED FOR PERSONAL USE

Conditions to be fulfilled:

1. Up to 100 average doses may be imported without any licence, provided it is part of passenger's luggage.

2. More than 100 doses are imported with licence. Applying in Form No: 12-A, 12-B.

3. The drug must be bonified personal use.

4. The quantity should be reasonable and covered by R.M.P prescription.

5. The drug must be declared to the Custom Collector if so directed.

IMPORT OF NEW DRUG

Conditions to be fulfilled:

1. Licence is required.

2. The licensee is required to provide the documents of standards of quality, purity and strength.

IMPORT OF DRUGS WITHOUT LICENCE (SCHEDULE-D DRUGS)

The following classes of drugs are imported without licence,

1. Substance not used for medicinal purpose.

2. Drugs in schedule C_1 required for manufacture and not for medicinal use. Importer should be holding licence for manufacture of schedule C/C_1.

3. Substances which are both drugs and foods such as,

   • Condensed/ powdered milk.   • Malt.

   • Lactose.   • Farex/cereal.   • Oats.

4. Pre-digested foods like Virol, Bovril, and Chicken essence.

5. Ginger, Pepper, Cumin, Cinnamon.

6. Drugs transit through India to foreign country.

OFFENCES AND PENALTIES

S.NO	OFFENCES	PENALTIES
1.	Import of spurious or adulterated drugs or import of drugs which involves risk to human beings or animals or drug not having claimed therapeutic values.	3 years imprisonment and Rs 5000/- fine (first conviction).5 years imprisonment and Rs 10,000/- fine or both (subsequent conviction).
2.	Contravention of the provision.	6 months imprisonment or Rs 500/- fine or both (first conviction). 1 year imprisonment and Rs 1000/- fine or both (subsequent conviction)

3.5 MANUFACTURING

TYPES OF MANUFACTURING LICENCES

1. For manufacture of other than Schedule C/C_1 and X drugs:

- Own premises.
- Loan licence.
- Repackaging licence.

2. For manufacture of only Schedule C/C_1 drugs:

- Own premises.
- Loan licence.

3. For manufacture of Schedule X drugs:

- Own premises.

4. For manufacture of Schedule C/C_1 and Schedule X drugs:

- Own premises.

FORMS

The different types of licences with corresponding form number and various fees is given in the following table,

S.no	Types of Licences	A	B	C	D	E
1.	Manufacture of other than C/C_1 and X with own premises.	24	25	400	100	50
2.	Manufacture of other than C/C_1 and X with loan premises.	24-A	25-A	200	100	50
3.	Repackaging of other than C/C_1 and X	24-B	25-B	80	20	10
4.	Manufacture of C/C_1 but not X with own premises.	27	28	600	400	200
5.	Manufacture of C/C_1 but not X with loan premises.	27-A	28-A	600	400	200
6.	Manufacture of X with own premises.	27-B	28-B	600	400	200
7.	Manufacture of C/C_1 and X with own premises.	27-B	28-B	1200	400	200
8.	Manufacture of Ayurvedic, Siddha, Unani.	24-D	25-D	60	-	60
9.	Manufacture of Ayurvedic, Siddha, Unani on loan licence.	25-E	25-E	30	-	30

In the above table, codes used as below

A = Form No for application   B = Form No to issue licence

C = Application fees   C = Inspecti-on fees

D = Renewal fees

PROHIBITION OF MANUFACTURE

1. Any drug which is not standard quality or is misbranded, adulterated or spurious.

2. Ant patent or proprietary medicine whose formula is not disclosed on the label or container.

3. Any drug which claims to prevent, cure or mitigate any disease specified in schedule J.

4. Any drug in contravention of this Act or Rules thereunder.

5. Any drug which has been manufactured in contravention of the provision of this Act or Rules.

6. Drugs which are likely to involve any risk to human being or animals.

7. Drug with no claimed therapeutic value.

MANUFACTURING OF DRUGS OTHER THAN THOSE SPECIFIED IN SCHEDULE C/C₁ AND SCHEDULE X

Procedure:

A licence is obtained from licensing authority (Foods and Drugs Control Administration) on application in prescribed Form No: 24 with prescribed fees (Rs 400, 100).

If the conditions are fulfilled, then licence is issued in a prescribed Form No: 25.

There are two types of conditions for all manufacturing licence. Conditions which are to be satisfied before a licence is granted and conditions which are to be complied with after a licence is granted.

Conditions (General):

1. The factory premises shall comply with the conditions laid down in the schedule M (space, premises, equipments and plants).

2. The manufacture shall be conducted under active supervision/ direction of *Competent Technical Staff.*

3. Adequate facilities for testing should be provided and it should be separate from manufacturing unit with an independent of department.

4. Adequate facilities for storage of drugs.

5. Licensee must allow an Inspector to inspect the premises, check the record and to take the sample.

6. Licensee must display the licence on the premises and produce it when asked for.

7. If any changes in the premise, plant or staff, it should be informed to the Authority.

8. Licensee must pay fees and get endorsement on the licence if the licensee wishes to manufacture any additional product.

9. Records of testing and manufacture (Sch-U) should be maintained at least for 2 years from the date of expiry of drugs and for 5 years in case of other drugs.

10. Licensee must provide samples to the Authority.

11. Licensee must furnish the data of stability of drug if demanded.

12. Licensee must provide any additional requirement as directed by the Authority.

13. Inspection book must be maintained.

14. The licensee shall comply with the requirements of "Good Manufacturing Practice".

15. The licensee shall maintain reference sample from each batch of the drugs manufactured, in a quantity which at least twice the quantity of the drug required to conduct all tests performed.

16. A statement of sales affected must be forwarded to the Authority every 3 months.

17. Accounts of production should be recorded and maintained for 5 years or 1 year after the date of expiry whichever later.

MANUFACTURE OF SCHEDULE C/C$_1$ (BIOLOGICALS)

A licence is obtained from licensing authority (Foods and Drugs Control Administration) on application in prescribed Form No: 27 with prescribed fees (Rs 600, 400).

If the conditions are fulfilled, then licence is issued in a prescribed Form No: 28.

Conditions:

The general conditions (1-17) applicable to other than Schedule C/C$_1$ and Schedule X are also applicable to manufacture of Schedule C/C$_1$.

Special conditions for Biologicals

1. All Schedule C drugs must be issued in previously sterilized, sealed glass of other suitable containers.

2. All the containers should comply with Schedule F/F$_1$.

3. The drug must comply with standards (strength, quality and purity) specified in Schedule F.

4. Some classes of substance should be tested for the absence of living aerobic and anaerobic micro-organisms.

   Ex: sera, bacterial vaccines, insulin etc.

5. Serum should be tested for freedom from abnormal toxicity.

6. Solution for parentral administration in dose of 10ml or more should be tested for freedom from pyrogens.

7. Multidose containers for liquids should contain preservatives to prevent growth of micro-organisms.

8. There should be separate laboratories culture and manipulation of spore bearing pathogens.

9. Sterility testing should be done.

10. Manufacturing of Schedule C/C$_1$ meant for animals should be carried out under supervision of Veterinary Science graduate with 4 years experience.

MANUFACTURE OF LARGE VOLUME PARENTRALS

Large volume parentrals means the sterile solutions intended for parentral administration with a volume of 100ml or more including anticoagulant solution in one container of the finished dosage form intended for single use.

Conditions:

The following are the additional conditions other than those (1-10) applicable to manufacture of Schedule C/C$_1$.

1. Provide and maintain adequate staff, premises, plant for manufacture and storage.

2. Separate laboratories, utensils and apparatus required for and manipulation of micro-organisms, not being used for any other purpose.

3. Maintain records as per Schedule U.

MANUFACTURE OF SCHEDULE-X DRUGS

Procedure:

A licence is obtained from licensing authority (Foods and Drugs Control Administration) on application in prescribed Form No: 27-B with prescribed fees (Rs 800, 100).

If the conditions are fulfilled, then licence is issued in a prescribed Form No: 28-B.

Conditions:

The general conditions (1-17) applicable to other than Schedule C/C$_1$ and Schedule X are also applicable to the manufacture of Schedule X.

Special Conditions:

1. Account of all transactions regarding manufacture should be maintained in a serially bound and paged register as follows. This should be preserved for 5 years.

    a) Accounts of drug used in manufacture.

- Date of issue.
- Name of the drug.
- Opening balance.
- Quantity received.
- Quantity used
- Balance quantity.
- Signature.

b) Account of production.

- Date of manufacture.
- Name of drug.
- Batch number.
- Quantity of raw material.
- Anticipated yield- actual yield.
- Wastage.
- Quantity of manufactured drug.

c) Account of manufactured drug.

- Date of manufacture.
- Name of the drug.
- Batch number.
- Opening balance.
- Quantity manufactured.
- Quantity sold.
- Name of purchaser.
- Balance quantity.

2. Manufacturer is required to send the copies of invoice of sale of drugs to licensing authority every 3 months.

3. The licensee should store Schedule-X drug in bulk form and when required for manufacture it should be kept in a separate place under direct custody of a responsible person.

4. Preparations should be labelled as X_{RX} (red ink).

5. No Schedule-X drugs should be supplied by the way of physician samples.

6. Drugs specified in Schedule-X shall be marketed in packaging not exceeding,

   •100 Unit dose- Tablet/Capsules.

   •300ml- Oral liquid.

   •5ml- Injection.

MANUFACTURING UNDER LOAN LICENCE

Loan Licence is given to a person (applicant) who does not have his own arrangements (factory) for manufacturing but wishes to avail the manufacturing facilities owned by another licensee.

In case of allopathic drugs the loan licences are issued for drug other than those specified in Schedule-X i.e.

• Drugs other than those specified in Schedule C/C₁ and Schedule-X.

• Drugs specified in Schedule C/C₁.

Procedure:

A licence is obtained from licensing authority (Foods and Drugs Control Administration) on application in prescribed Form No: 24-A, 27-A with prescribed fees (Rs 200, 100-600, 400).

If the conditions are fulfilled, then licence is issued in a prescribed Form No: 25-A, 28-A.

Conditions:

The general conditions (1-17) applicable to other than Schedule C/C₁ and Schedule X are also applicable to the manufacturing of drugs other than those specified in Schedule C/C$_1$ and Schedule-X, under Loan Licence.

In addition to general conditions (1-17), if loan licensee wishes to manufacture biological products (C/C$_1$) then he has to comply with special conditions for biological (1-9).

Additional conditions:

1. Application must be supported by the parent firm.

2. Drug inspector inspects the premises of parent firm and checks and assesses the spare capacity.

3. Loan licensee is required to test each batch of raw materials and finished products.

4. Records of testing should be maintained for 5 years or 2 years in case of expiry drugs from such date.

5. If the licence of parent firm is cancelled or suspended, the loan licence will also be deemed to be suspended or cancelled.

6. Patent or proprietary medicines should contain the constituent ingredients in therapeutic or prophylactic quantities.

7. Patent medicines must be safe for use in the context of vehicle and additives.

8. The ingredients and their quantities must have therapeutic justification,

9. The production must be supervised by competent person of loan licensee.

REPACKAGING LICENCES

Process of breaking up any drug from its bulk container into small packages and labelling with a view to their sale and distribution is done under repackaging licence.

Repackaging licence is granted for drug other than those specified in Schedule C/C$_1$ and Schedule-X.

Procedure:

A licence is obtained from licensing authority (Foods and Drugs Control Administration) on application in prescribed Form No: 24-B with prescribed fees (Rs 80, 20).

If the conditions are fulfilled, then licence is issued in a prescribed Form No: 25-B.

Conditions:

1. Adequate space and equipment should be provided. Repackaging must be carried out under hygienic conditions.

2. Repackaging should be supervised by competent person.

3. Adequate arrangement for analysis of raw materials and repacked drugs.

4. Maintain record of analysis for at least 3 years from the date of manufacture, 3 months for expiry dated drug from such date.

5. Adequate space for storage of drugs should be provided.

6. Licensee should allow an Inspector to inspect the premises, records and take samples of drug.

7. The licence should be displayed on the premises.

8. Factory premises must comply with the conditions prescribed in Schedule M.

9. If any change in the competent staff, immediately inform the authority.

10. Label should bear R.P.G Licence number.

OFFENCES AND PENALTIES

S.No	OFFENCES	PENALTIES
1.	Manufacture of adulterated or spurious drugs which are likely to cause death.	5 year to life time imprisonment and not less than Rs 10,000/- fine.
2.	Manufacture of drug without licence.	1-3 years imprisonment and Rs 5000/- fine (1st conviction).2-6 years imprisonment and Rs 10,000/- fine (subsequent conviction).
3.	Manufacture of any drug in contravention to the provision of the Act.	1-2 years imprisonment with fine.
4.	Person who do not maintain the record or disclose the information.	1 year imprisonment and/or Rs 1000/- fine.
5.	Manufacturer who gives false warranty, that drugs do not contravene any provision of the Act.	1 year imprisonment and/or Rs 500/- fine.
6.	Anyone who uses analytical report for advertising purpose.	Rs 500/- fine (1st conviction). 10 years imprisonment or fine or both (subsequent conviction).

3.6 SALES

TYPES OF SALES LICENCE

For the sale of allopathic drugs different types of sales licence are available as follows.

1. **Whole sale licence**

   - Drugs other than those specified in Schedule C/C$_1$ and Schedule-X.

- Drugs specified in Schedule C/C_1.

- Drugs specified in Schedule-X.

2. **Retail sale licence**

a) *General licence:*

- Drugs other than those specified in Schedule C/C_1 and Schedule-X.

- Drugs specified in Schedule C/C_1.

- Drugs specified in Schedule-X.

b) *Restricted licence:*

- Drugs other than those specified in Schedule C/C_1 and Schedule-X.

- Drugs specified in Schedule C/C_1.

3. **Sale from motor vehicle (vendor)**

- Drugs other than those specified in Schedule C/C_1 and Schedule-X.

- Drugs specified in Schedule C/C_1.

FORMS

The different types of licences with corresponding Form number and various fees is given in the following table

S.no	Types of Licence	A	B	C
1.	Wholesale of other than those specified in Schedule C/C₁ and Schedule-X.	19	20-B	40
2.	Wholesale of drugs specified in Schedule C/C₁.	19-C	21-B	40
3.	Wholesale of drugs specified in Schedule-X.	19-C	20-G	40
4.	Retail sale of other than those specified in Schedule C/C₁ and Schedule-X.	19	20	40
5.	Retail sale of drugs specified in Schedule C/C₁.	19	21	40
6.	Retail sale of drugs specified in Schedule-X.	19-C	20-F	40
7.	Restricted retail sale of other than those specified in Schedule C/C₁ and Schedule-X.	19-A	20-A	40 OR 10
8.	Restricted retail sale of drugs specified in Schedule C/C₁.	19-A	21-A	40 OR 10
9.	Sales from motor vehicle of drugs other than Schedule C/C₁.	19-AA	20-BB	20
10.	Sales from motor vehicle of drugs specified in Schedule C/C₁.	19-AA	20-BB	20

In the above table, codes used as below

A = No's of Form for application
B = No's of Form to issue licence
C = Application fees

PROHIBITION OF SALE OR CERTAIN DRUGS AND COSMETICS

From such date as may be fixed by the State Government by notification in the Official Gazette in this behalf, no person shall himself or by any other person on his behalf-

a) Sell, or stock or exhibit or offer for sale, or distribute –

i.   Any drug which is not of a standard quality, or is misbranded, adulterated or spurious.

ii.   Any cosmetic which is not of a standard quality or is misbranded or spurious.

iii.   Any patent or proprietary medicine, unless there is displayed in the prescribed manner on the label or container thereof the true formula or list of active ingredients contained in it together with the quantities, thereof

iv.   Any drug which by means of any statement design or device accompanying it or by any other means, purports or claims to prevent, cure or mitigate any such disease or ailment, or to have any such other effect as may be prescribed.

v.   Any cosmetic containing any ingredient, which may render it unsafe or harmful for use under the directions, indicated or recommended.

vi.   Any drug or cosmetic in contravention of any of the provisions of this Chapter or any rule made there under.

b) Sell or stock or exhibit or offer for sale, or distribute any drug or cosmetic which has been imported or manufactured in contravention of any of the provisions of this Act or any rule made there under.

c) Sell, or stock or exhibit or offer for sale, or distribute any drug or cosmetic, except under, and in accordance with the conditions of, a licence issued for such purpose under this Chapter.

Provided that nothing in this section shall apply to the manufacture, subject to prescribed conditions, of small quantities of any drug for the purpose of examination, test or analysis.

Provided further that the Central Government may, after consultation with the Board by notification in the Official Gazette, permit, subject to any conditions specified in the notification, the sale, stocking or exhibiting or offering for sale or distribution of any drug or class of drugs not being of standard quality.

A. WHOLESALE

CONDITIONS FOR THE WHOLESALE OF BIOLOGICALS (SCHEDULE C/C₁)

Procedure:

A licence is obtained from licensing authority (Foods and Drugs Control Administration) on application in prescribed Form No: 19 with prescribed fees (Rs 40).

If the conditions are fulfilled, then licence is issued in a prescribed Form No: 21-B.

Conditions:

1. Premises not less than $10m^2$, equipped with the facilities for proper storage of drugs.

2. Precaution should be taken while storing the drugs.

3. The drugs should be sold to only those people who are licensed to retail them.

4. Premises should be in charge of *Competent Person*.

5. Exemptions to the sale of drugs to,

   • Hospital institutes.

   • Medical institutes.

   • Educational institutes.

   • Research institutes.

- Government authorities.
- Manufacturers of Oil, Beverages and Confectionery.

6. Licensee should obtain the permission for any additional category of sale.

7. Records of purchase and sale should be maintained under the following heading,

   - Date of purchase and sale.
   - Name/ Address of firm from whom purchased and to whom sold.
   - Names, quantities and batch no. of drugs.
   - Names of manufacturers.

8. Records should be preserved for 3 years from the date of sale.

9. Licence should be displayed on the premises.

CONDITION FOR WHOLESALE OF DRUGS OTHER THAN THOSE SPECIFIED IN SCHEDULE C/C₁AND SCHEDULE-X

Procedure:

A licence is obtained from licensing authority (Foods and Drugs Control Administration) on application in prescribed Form No: 19 with prescribed fees (Rs 40).

If the conditions are fulfilled, then licence is issued in a prescribed Form No: 20-B.

Conditions:

The conditions (1-9) applicable to wholesale of Schedule C/C₁ are also applicable to the wholesale of drugs other than those specified in Schedule C/C₁ and Schedule-X along with the following additional conditions.

1. The licensee should comply with the provisions of drugs and cosmetics Act- 1940 and rules there under.

2. The compounding is made by or under the direct or personal supervision of a qualified person.

CONDITIONS FOR THE WHOLESALE OF SCHEDULE-X DRUGS

Procedure:

A licence is obtained from licensing authority (Foods and Drugs Control Administration) on application in prescribed Form No: 19-C with prescribed fees (Rs 40).

If the conditions are fulfilled, then licence is issued in a prescribed Form No: 20-G.

Conditions:

The conditions (1-9) applicable to wholesale of Schedule C/C$_1$ and wholesale of drugs other than those specified in Schedule C/C$_1$ and Schedule-X (1-2) are also applicable to the wholesale of Schedule-X drugs along with the following additional condition.

1. The licensee should forward the copies of invoice of sales made by the retail dealer to the licensing authority.

B. RETAIL SALE

For retail sale two types of licence are issued,

1. General licence.

2. Restricted licence.

GENERAL LICENCE

General licences are granted to the person who have the premises for the business and who engage the service of a qualified person to supervise the sale and do compounding and dispensing.

General licence for the retail sale of the drug are issued for the following categories of drugs,

1. Drugs other than those specified in Schedule C/C$_1$ and Schedule-X.

2. Drugs specified in Schedule C/C$_1$.

3. Drugs specified in Schedule-X.

Conditions:

1. Adequate premises of 10m² and equipped with adequate facilities for storage and under the incharge of qualified person to supervise the sale.

2. The licensee should meet the requirements prescribed in Schedule-N.

3. The licensee should obtain the permission of the licensing authority for any additional sales.

4. All registers and records should be maintained for 2 years,

5. Licensee should allow the Inspector to inspect the premises, register and records.

6. The licensing authority must be informed if there is any change in the qualified person.

7. Precautions should be taken in the storage of biological products (Sch C/C$_1$).

8. The licence should be displayed at a prominent place in the premises.

9. The licensee should comply with the provisions of the Drugs and Cosmetics Act and Rules.

10. Drugs should be purchased only from the licensed dealer of manufacturer.

11. The Inspection book should be maintained.

12. Do not stock or sell expired drugs.

13. Drugs should be sold only to licence or prescription holder.

14. No drugs intended for Physician samples, E.S.I.S, Central government Health Service etc shall be stocked or sold.

15. In case of loose supply from the main container, the label should contain the following details,

- Name of the drug.

- Quantity supplied.

- Name/address of dealer.

- Storage conditions.

16. Veterinary products stored separately and labelled as "Not for Human Use- for treatment of animal only".

17. If drug is dispensed after compounding, it shall be recorded in the prescription register.

18. The supply of drugs other than those specified in Schedule-X on prescription shall be recorded in prescription register. The following particulars shall be entered.

- Serial No

- Date of supply.

- Name/address of prescriber.

- Name/address of patient or owner of animal.

- Name/quantity of drug.

- In case of schedule-C or H, name of manufacturer, batch no, date of expiry etc.

- Signature of qualified person.

19. In place of prescription register, the licensee shall maintain carbon copies of Cash/Credits memos which shall contain the following,

- Name, address and sale licence no of the dealer.

- Serial no of the Cash/Credit memos.

- Name/quantity of drug supplied.

20. Records of purchase of drug shall be maintained with following particulars,

- Date of purchase.

- Name/address of the person from whom purchased and licence no held.

- Name/quantity of drug with batch no.

- Name of manufacturer.

- Purchase bill shall be maintained.

RESTRICTED LICENCE

Restricted licence is granted to those dealers who do not engage the service of qualified person and only deal with such class of drugs whose sale can be effected without qualified person and vendors do not have fixed premises.

Restricted licences for retail sale are issued for only specified categories of the drugs as follows.

1. A licence in Form no: 21-A (restricted biologicals) shall not be granted for drugs specified in Schedule C and valid only for specified C_1 drugs.

2. Other than those specified in Schedule C/C$_1$ and Schedule-X.

3. Restricted licence may also be issued to a travelling agent of a firm for the special purpose of distribution of the medical practitioners or dealers, for supply of biological.

Conditions:

1. The licensee shall deal with only such drugs that can be sold without supervision of qualified person.

2. If licensee is vendor, he should buy drugs only from fixed dealer which is specified in the licence.

3. Adequate precautions for preserving the properties of drug should be taken.

4. The licence should be prominently in the premises. In case of vendor it should remain with the person.

5. The drugs should be sold in their original containers.

6. Drugs should be purchased only from a duly licensed dealer of manufacturer.

7. The licensee should comply with the provisions of the Drug and Cosmetic Act and Rules.

C. MOTOR-VEHICLE

Sale of drugs from motor-vehicle is a part of wholesale. There are 2 types of licences issued for this purpose.

1. Licence for sale of drugs other than those specified in Schedule C/C$_1$.

2. Licence for sale of drugs specified in Schedule C/C$_1$.

Conditions:

1. The licence should be displayed on the prominent part of the vehicle.

2. The licensee should comply with the provisions of the Drug and Cosmetic Act and Rules.

3. Drugs should be purchased from the licensed dealer or manufacturer.

4. The drugs should be sold only to the person holding licence.

5. Licensing authority should be informed.

6. Precaution for storage should be taken.

The conditions (1-5) are applicable for the sale of drugs other than those specified in Schedule C/C$_1$ and condition (1, 2, 3, 5 and 6) are applicable to the sale of drugs specified in Schedule C/C$_1$.

SPECIAL PROVISIONS

Dispensing of compounded drugs:

1. Drugs should be compounded by the qualified person.

2. It should be recorded in the register under the following headings.

    • Serial number.

    • Name/address of the prescriber.

    • Name/address of patient or owner of animals.

    • If Schedule C or H drugs, name of the manufacturer, batch number and date of expiry.

    • Signature of the qualified person.

    • In case of refill prescription, serial number, date of supply, quantity supplied.

    • Schedule H drugs should not be dispensed more than twice unless specified.

Supply of Schedule C/C$_1$ drugs:

The records should have the following details.

1. Serial number.

2. Date of supply.

3. Name/address of purchaser.

4. Name /quantity of drugs.

5. Name of manufacturer, batch no, date of expiry.

6. Signature of qualified person.

Supply of Schedule H and X drugs:

1. Retailed only on RMP prescription.

2. Do not dispense more than once unless specified.

3. No substitutions should be made while dispensing.

4. In case of Schedule-X drugs, the prescription should be in duplicate and following particulars should be entered in the register,

- Date of supply and opening and closing stock.

- Name of drug, its manufacturer's name and batch number.

- Name/address of purchaser.

- Date of prescription and name/address of RMP.

- Signature of qualified person.

Storage of Schedule-X drugs:

1. Stored under lock and key in a cupboard reserved solely for the storage of these substances.

2. Separate storage from the remainder of the premises.

3. Only responsible person has access.

Storage of Veterinary Medicines:

1. It should be stored in a separate cupboard labelled as "Not for Human Use- For Treatment of Animals Only".

2. Portion of the premises separated from the remainder of the premises to which customers are not permitted to have access.

QUALIFIED PERSON

Qualified person who supervises the sale of drugs is the one with the following qualifications.

- Person holding a Diploma or Degree in Pharmacy or Pharmaceutical chemistry.

- Registered Pharmacist.

- Person with 4 years of experience before 31/12/1969.

OFFENCES AND PENALTIES

S.no	OFFENCES	PENALTIES
1.	Selling adulterated or spurious drugs or drugs that are likely to cause death.	5 years to lifetime imprisonment and Rs 10,000/- fine (1st conviction).10 years imprisonment or Rs 20,000/- fine or both (subsequent conviction).
2.	Sales of adulterated drugs that do not cause death or sale of drugs without valid licence.	1-3 years imprisonment and Rs 5000/- fine (1st conviction). 2-6 years imprisonment and Rs10,000/- fine (subsequent conviction).
3.	Sale of any drug in contravention of the provision of the Act.	1-2 years imprisonment and fine (1st conviction).2-4 years imprisonment and/or Rs 5000/- fine (subsequent conviction).
4.	Records not maintained or information not disclosed.	3 years imprisonment and/or Rs 1000/- fine (1st conviction).
5.	False warranty that drugs do not contravene any provision of the Act.	1 year imprisonment or Rs 500/- fine (1st conviction). 2 years imprisonment and/or fine (subsequent conviction).
6.	Use of analytical report for advertisement.	Rs 500/- fine (1st conviction). 10 years imprisonment and/or fine (subsequent conviction).

DISPOSAL OF EXPIRED DRUGS

1. Instead of returning the drugs to the manufacturer, the expired drugs should be destroyed at the premises of the licensee holding such drugs.

2. Expired drugs are not to be destroyed at the premises of the licensee within 03 months from the expiry date.

DISPOSAL OF DRUGS IF LICENCE IS CANCELLED

1. If the licensee wishes to dispose the drugs in his possession in the premises in respect of which the licence has been cancelled, he should apply in writing to the licensing authority giving the following particulars.

    • Name and address of the person to whom the drugs are proposed to be sold and his licence number.

    • Name of drugs, their quantities, batch number, name/address of manufacturer and expiry date.

2. The licensing authority, after examination of the particulars furnished and after Inspection by an Inspector, grants the necessary permission for the disposal.

3.7 LABELLING - PACKAGING

LIST OF DRUGS PERTAININBG TO DIFFERENT SCHEDULES

SCHEDULE C DRUGS (BIOLOGICAL PARENTRAL):

1. Sera
2. Solution of serum proteins intended for injection.
3. Vaccines for parentral injections.
4. Toxins.
5. Antigen.
6. Antitoxins.
7. Neo-arsphenamine and analogous substances used for the specific treatment of
8. Infective diseases.
9. Insulin.
10. Pituitary (Posterior Lobe) Extract.
11. Adrenaline and Solutions of Salts of Adrenaline.

12. Antibiotics and preparations thereof in a form to be administered parenterally.

13. Any other preparation which is meant for parentral administration as such or after being made up with a solvent or medium or any other sterile product and which requires to be stored in a refrigerator; or does not require to be stored in a refrigerator.

14. Sterilized surgical ligature and sterilized surgical suture.

15. Bacteriophages.

16. Ophthalmic preparations.

Sterile Disposable Devices for single use only

SCHEDULE C₁ DRUGS (BIOLOGICAL NON-PARENTRAL):

1. Drugs belonging to the Digitalis groups and preparations containing drugs belonging to the Digitalis group not in a form to be administered parentally.

2. Ergot and preparations containing Ergot not in a form to be administered parentally.

3. Adrenaline and preparations containing Adrenaline not in a form to be administered parenterally.

4. Fish Liver Oil and preparations containing Fish Liver Oil.

5. Vitamins and preparations containing any vitamins not in a form to be administered parenterally.

6. Liver extract and preparations containing liver extract not in a form to be administered parenterally.

7. Hormones and preparations containing Hormones not in a form to be administered parenterally.

8. Vaccine not in a form to be administered parenterally.

9. Antibiotics and preparations thereof not in a form to be administered parenterally.

10. In-vitro Blood Grouping Sera.

11. In-vitro diagnostic Devices for HIV, HbsAg and HCV.

SCHEDULE G DRUGS:

1. Aminopterin
2. L-Asparaginase
3. Bleomycin
4. Busulphan; its salts
5. Carbutamide
6. Chlorambucil;its salts
7. Chlorothiazide and other derivatives of 1, 2, 4 benzothiadrazine
8. Chlorpropamide; its salts
9. Chlorthalidone and other derivatives of Chlorobenzene compound.
10. Cis-Platin
11. Cyclophosphamide; its salts
12. Cytarabine
13. Daunorubicin
14. Di-Isopropyl Eluorophosphate
15. Disodium Stilboestrol Diphosphate
16. Doxorubicin Hydrochloride
17. Ethacrynic acid, its salts
18. Ethosuximide
19. Glibenclamide
20. Hydantoin; its salts, its derivatives, their salts
21. Hydroxyurea
22. Insulin, all types
23. Lomustine Hydrochloride

24. Mannomustine; its salts

25. Mercaptopurine; its salts

26. Metformin; its salts

27. Methsuximide

28. Mustine, its salts

29. Paramethadione

30. Phenacemide

SCHEDULE H (PRESCRIPTION DRUGS):

1. Acebutolol Hydrochloride

2. Aclarubicin Inj

3. Actilyse

4. Acyclovir

5. Barbituric acid, its salts, derivative of

6. Barbituric acid, their salts

7. Bacampicillin

8. Benserazide Hydrochloride

9. Captopril

10. Carbidopa

11. Carbocisteine

12. Carboplatin Injection

13. Danzol

14. Dapsone, its salts and derivatives

15. Desogestrol

16. Dextranomer

17. Econozole

18. Enalapril Maleate

19. Enfenamic Acid
20. Epinephrine, its salts
21. Flurazepam
22. Flurbiprofen
23. Glucagon
24. Glycopyrrolate
25. Heparin
26. Hepatitis B. Vaccine
27. Ketamine Hydrochloride
28. Ketoconazole Acetate
29. LevodopA
30. Nalidixic Acid
31. Naproxen

SCHEDULE-J (INCURABLE DISEASES):

1. AIDS
2. Angina Pectoris
3. Appendicitis
4. Arteriosclerosis
5. Baldness
6. Blindness
7. Bronchial Asthma
8. Cancer and Benign tumour
9. Cataract
10. Change in colour of the hair and growth of new hair.
11. Change of Foetal sex by drugs.
12. Congenital malformations

13. Deafness

14. Diabetes

15. Diseases and disorders of uterus.

16. Epileptic-fits and psychiatric disorders

17. Encephalitis

18. Fairness of the skin

19. Form, structure of breast

20. Gangrene

21. Genetic disorders

22. Glaucoma

23. Goitre

24. Hernia

25. High/low Blood Pressure

SCHEDULE-O (STANDARD FOR DISINFECTANT FLUIDS):

1. The disinfectants shall be classified as follows: -

    a) Black fluids.

    b) White fluids.

Black fluids:

These shall be homogeneous dark brown solution of coal tar acid or similar acids derived from petroleum with or without hydrocarbon, and/or other phenolic compounds, and their derivatives and a suitable emulsifier.

White fluids:

These shall be finely dispersed homogeneous white to off-white emulsion consisting of coal tar acids or similar acids derived from petroleum, with or without hydrocarbons, and/or other phenolic compounds, and their derivatives.

2. *Gradation:* Each of the above classes of disinfectant fluids shall be graded on the basis of the minimum requirements in respect of, Rideal Walker (RW) Coefficient as follows,

Grade	Rideal Walker (RW) coefficient (minimum)
1.	18
2.	10
3.	05

3. *Type*: Each of the above grades of disinfectant fluids shall be stable in the range of temperature indicated against each type. –

Type Stable in the range of

a)   Normal- 15°C to 45°C.

b)   Winter- 5°C to 30°C.

4. *Requirements.* - All classes and grades of disinfectant fluids shall comply with the following requirements, namely

a) Stability after dilution: When tested by the method described hereinafter the disinfectant fluids shall be miscible with artificial hard water (for Black fluids) or with artificial sea water (for White fluids) in all proportion from 1 per cent to 5 per cent by volume, to give emulsion which shall not break or show more than traces of separation of either top or bottom oil when kept for 6 hours at 15°C to 45°C for Type (I) (Normal) and 5°C to 30°C for Type (II) (Winter).

b) *Germicidal Value:* Rideal Walker Coefficient – Black fluids and White fluids shall be used tested for determination of Rideal Walker Coefficient (R.W.Coefficient) by the method described hereinafter.

c) Storage: Disinfectant fluids of all classes shall be stored in mild steel, tinned mild steel or other suitable containers. These shall not be stored in containers made of galvanized iron.

d) Labelling: Subject to the other provisions in these rules, the label on the container shall state-

- The name of the product,

- The name and full address of the manufacturer,

- Grade, type, R.W. Coefficient of product,

- Date of manufacture,

- Quantity present in the container,

- Indications and mode of use, and

- Date up to which the product can be used.

SCHEDULE-P (LIFE PERIOD OD DRUGS):

S.no	NAME OF DRUGS	PERIOD (Months)	STORAGE CONDITION
1.	AMPICILLIN (Capsule, Dry Syrup, Injection)	24	COOL PLACE
2.	BACITRACIN (Tablet, Lozenges)	12	-
3.	CEPHALEXIN	24	COOL PLACE
4.	CHLORAMPHENICOL (Oral syrup)	36	-
5.	GRISEOFULVIN (Tablets)	36	-
6.	RIFAMPICIN (Capsule)	24	COOL PLACE
7.	INSULIN (Injection)	24	2-8° C, NOT TO FREEZE.
8.	VITAMIN-A (Injection)	24	-
9.	VITAMIN-B1 (Injection)	24	-
10.	ADRENALINE (Injection)	12	COOL PLACE

SECHEDULE-W (DRUGS MARKETED UNDER GENERIC NAMES):

1. Analgin.
2. Aspirin and its salts.
3. Chlorpromazine and its salts.
4. Ferrous sulphate.
5. Piperazine and its salts.

SCHEDULE-X DRUGS (NARCOTIC AND PSYCHOTROPIC SUBSTANCES):

1. Amobarbital
2. Amphetamina
3. Methylphenidate
4. Barbital
5. Methylphenobarbital
6. Cyclobarbital
7. Pentobarbital
8. Dexamphetamine
9. Phencyclidine
10. Ethclorvynol
11. Phenmetrazine
12. Glutethimide
13. Meprobamate
14. Secobarbital
15. Methamphetamine

LIST OF PERMITTED COLOURS

1. *Natural colours:*

   a) Annatto.

   b) Carotene.

   c) Red oxide of iron.

   d) Titanium dioxide.

   e) Cochineal.

   f) Chlorophyll.

   g) Yellow oxide of iron.

2. *Artificial colours:*

   a) Caramel.

   b) Riboflavin.

3. *Coal tar colours:*

   a) Green- Quinazarin green SS, Alizarincyanine green SS.

   b) Yellow- Tartrazine, Sunset yellow FCF.

   c) Red- Erythrosine, Sudan-III.

   d) Blue- Indigo carmine, Brilliant blue FCF.

   e) Violet- Alizurol purple SS.

   f) Orange- Orange G.

   g) Brown- Resorcin brown.

   h) Black- Naphthol blue black.

Schedule F (provisions applicable to Vaccines, Toxins, Antigens and Sera):

1. *Vaccines:*

   a) Supervised by competent expert in bacteriology.

   b) Named with micro-organism followed by the word "vaccine".

c) Keep the records of the origin property and characteristics of the culture.

d) Label shall indicate the following,

- Number of micro-organism per cubic centimetre.

- Weight of dried substance per cubic centimetre.

e) General test for sterility should be done.

2. *Toxins:*

a) Label should clearly indicate Schick Test Toxin.

b) Undiluted or diluted- Schick control.

c) Potency test.

d) Sterility test.

e) Toxicity test.

3. *Sera:*

a) Supervised by competent expert in bacteriology.

b) Animal house should be at distance.

c) Adequate number of efficient sterilizers must be provided.

d) Only healthy and uninfected animals must be used.

e) Labelled with proper name,

Ex: Anti Meningococcus serum.

f) Amount expressed in cubic centimetre.

g) The culture used shall be opened to inspection.

h) Maintain the quality and strength.

i) Unit of standardisation.

3.8 MANNER OF LABELLING

1. Subject to the other provisions of these rules, the following particulars shall be either printed or written in indelible ink and shall appear in a conspicuous manner on the label of the innermost container of any drug and on every other covering which the container is packed, namely

i.   The name of the drug

For this purpose, the proper name of the drug shall be printed or written in a more conspicuous manner than the trade name, if any, which shall be shown immediately after or under the proper name and shall be,

a) for drugs included in the Schedule F or Schedule F (1), the name given therein

b) for drugs included in the India Pharmacopoeia or the official pharmacopoeia and official compendia of drug standards prescribed in the rule 124, the name or synonym specified in the respective official pharmacopoeias and official compendia of drug standards followed by the letters 'I.P., or, as the case may be, by the recognized abbreviations of the respective official pharmacopoeias and official compendia of drug standards;

c) for drugs included in the National Formulary of India, the name or synonym specified therein followed by the letters 'N.F.I.';

d) for other drugs, the international non-proprietary name, if any, published by the World Health Organisation or where an international non-proprietary name is not published, the name descriptive of the true nature or origin of the substance;

ii. A correct statement of the net content in terms of weight, measure, volume, number of units of contents, number of units of activity, as the case may be, and the weight, measure and volume shall be expressed in Metric system.

iii. The content of active ingredients.

This shall be expressed as,

a) For oral liquid preparations in terms of the content per single dose being indicated in 5 millilitres

b) For liquid parentral preparations ready for administration in terms of 1 millilitres or percentage by volume or per dose in the case of single dose container.

c) For drugs in solid form intended for parentral administration, in terms of units or weight per milligram or gram;

d) For tablets, capsules, pills and the like, in terms of the content in each tablet, capsule, pill or other unit, as the case may be;

e) For other preparations, in terms of percentage by weight or volume or in terms of unit age per gram or millilitre, as the case may be.

iv.   The name of the manufacturer and the address of the premises of the manufacturer where the drug has been manufactured.

Provided that of the drug is contained in an ampoule or a similar small container, it shall be enough if only the name of the manufacturer and his principal place of manufacture are shown;

v.   A distinctive batch number, that is to say, the number by reference to which details of manufacture of the particular batch from which the substance in the container is taken are recorded and are available for inspection, the figure representing the batch number being preceded by the words 'Batch No.' or 'B. No.' or 'Batch' or 'Lot No.' or 'Lot'.

2. (i) The particulars to be printed or written on the label of a mechanical contraceptive shall be as specified in Schedule R.

(ii) The following particulars, in addition to those specified under sub-rule (i) shall be either printed or written in indelible ink and shall appear in a conspicuous manner on the label of the innermost container and on every other covering in which the container of a contraceptive, other than a mechanical contraceptive, is packed, namely

a) The date of manufacture;

b) The date up to which the contraceptive is expected to retain its properties;

c) The storage conditions necessary for preserving the properties of the contraceptive up to the date indicated in sub-clause (b) :

Provided that for oral contraceptives it shall be sufficient to display on the label of the container the date of manufacture only.

3. (i) The particulars prescribed in sub-rule (1) shall be printed or written in indelible ink either on the label borne by a container of vaccine lymph or on a label or wrapper affixed to any package in which the container is issued for sale. The said particulars shall be indelibly marked on the sealed container of surgical ligature or suture or printed or written in indelible ink on a label enclosed therein.

(ii) Nothing in these rules shall be deemed to require the labelling of any transparent cover or of any wrapper, case or other covering used solely for the purpose of packing, transport or delivery.

4. Where be any provision of these rules any particulars are required to be displayed on a label on the container, such particulars may, instead of being displayed on a label, be etched, painted or otherwise indelibly marked on the container :

Provided that, except where otherwise provided in these rules, the name of the drug or any distinctive letters intended to refer to the drug shall not be etched, painted or otherwise indelibly marked on any glass container other than ampoules.

LABELLING OF MEDICINES

1. The container of a medicine for internal use shall—

a)   if it contains a substance specified in Schedule G, be labelled with the words 'Caution: it is dangerous to take this preparation except under medical supervision' – conspicuously printed and surrounded by a line within which there shall be no other words;

b)   if it contains a substance specified in Schedule H be labelled with the symbol Rx and conspicuously displayed on the left top corner of the label and be also labelled with the following words:

Schedule H drug- 'Warning: To be sold by retail on the prescription of a Registered Medical Practitioner only'

c)   If it contains a substance specified in Schedule H, and comes within the purview of the Narcotic Drugs and Psychotropic Substances Act, 1985 be labelled with the symbol NRx which shall be in red and conspicuously displayed on the left top corner of the label, and be also labelled with the following words:

Schedule H drug -"*Warning:* To be sold by retail on the prescription of a Registered Medical Practitioner only."

d)   If it contains a substance specified in Schedule X, be labelled with the symbol XRx which shall be in red conspicuously displayed on the left top corner of the label and be also labelled with the words : -

Schedule X drug -"*Warning:* To be sold by retail on the prescription of a Registered Medical Practitioner only."

2.   The container of an embrocation, liniment, lotion, 2[ointment, antiseptic cream,] liquid antiseptic or other liquid medicine for external application shall be labelled with the word in capital 'For External use only.'

3.   The container of a medicine made up ready only for treatment of an animal shall be labelled conspicuously with the words 'Not for human use; for animal treatment only' and shall bear a symbol depicting the head of a domestic animal.

4.   The container of a medicine prepared for treatment of human ailments shall if the medicine contains industrial methylated spirit, indicate this fact on the label and be labelled with the words : "For External Use only".

5.   Substances specified in Schedule X in bulk form shall bear a label wherein they symbol as specified in sub-rule (1) shall be given conspicuously in red letters.

NON-STERILE SURGICAL LIGATURE AND SUTURE

1.   Every container of, and wrapper enclosing surgical ligature or suture other than a ligature or suture offered or intended to be offered for sale as sterile, shall bear a label on which are printed

or written in a conspicuous manner in indelible red ink the words "Non-sterile surgical ligature (suture) – not be used for operations upon the human body unless efficiently sterilized".

2. The name and address of the manufacturer shall be printed on the label of the container of a patent or proprietary medicine.

3. The true formula or list of the ingredients shall be printed or written in indelible ink on the outer label of every package containing patent or proprietary medicine.

USE OF LETTER I.P

The letters 'I.P' and recognized abbreviations of pharmacopoeias and official compendia of drug standards prescribed under these rules shall be entered on the label of the drug only for the purpose of indicating that the drug is in accordance with standards set out in the Indian Pharmacopoeia or in any such pharmacopoeia or official compendium of drug standards recognized under the Rules.

3.9 PACKING OF DRUGS

1. The pack sizes of drugs meant for retail sale shall be as prescribed in Schedule P-1 to these rules.

2. The pack sizes of drugs not covered by the Schedule P-1 shall be as given below, unless specified otherwise in Schedule P-1,

   i. The pack sizes for Tablets/Capsules shall be-

Where the number of Tablets (coated or uncoated)/Capsules (hard or soft gelatin) is less than 10, such packing shall be made by the integral number. For numbers above 10, the pack size of Tablets/Capsules shall contain multiples of 5.

   ii. The pack sizes for liquid Oral preparations shall be 30ml (paediatric only) 60ml/100 ml/200 ml/450 ml.

   iii. The pack sizes for Paediatric Oral Drops shall be 5 ml/10 ml/ 15 ml.

   iv. The pack sizes for Eye/Ear/Nasal drops shall be 3 ml/5 ml/10 ml.

v. The pack size for Eye Ointment shall be 3 gm/5 gm/ 10 gm.

Provided that the provisions of the pack sizes covered under this rule shall not apply to:

- Pack sizes or dosage forms not covered by the foregoing provisions of this rule.

- The imported formulations in finished form.

- Preparations intended for Veterinary use.

- Preparations intended for Export.

- Vitamins/Tonics/Cough Preparations/Antacids/Laxatives in Liquid Oral forms, Unit dose (including applicaps).

- Pack sizes of dosage form meant for retail sale to Hospitals, Registered Medic al practitioners, Nursing Homes.

- Physician's Samples.

- Pack sizes of large volume intravenous fluids.

Provided also that pack sizes of any of the new drug as and when approved by the Licensing Authority appointed under Rule 21 and if not covered under this rule, shall be examined for the purpose of approval with the specific justification by the said Licensing Authority.

Provided further that Oxytocin injection meant for sale shall be in single unit blister pack only.

PACKINGS OF DRUGS SPECIFIED IN SCHEDULE X

The drugs specified in Schedule X shall be marketed in packing not exceeding-

i.   100 unit doses in the case of tablets/capsules.

ii.   300ml in the case of oral liquid preparations.

iii. And 5 ml in the case of injections.

Provided that nothing in this rule shall apply to packing meant for use of a hospital or a dispensary subject to the conditions that-

i.   Such supplied are made by the manufacturers or distributors direct to the hospital/dispensaries; and

ii. Hospital packs shall not be supplied to a retain dealer or to a Registered Medical Practitioner.

3.10 SCHEDULE N

(List of minimum equipment for the efficient running of a pharmacy)

1. *Entrance:* The front of a pharmacy shall bear an inscription "Pharmacy" in front.

2. *Premises:*

   a)   The premises of a pharmacy shall be separated from rooms for private use. The premises shall be well built, dry, well lit and ventilated and of sufficient dimensions to allow the goods in stock especially medicaments and poisons to be kept in a clearly visible and appropriate manner.

   b)   The area of the section to be used as dispensing department shall be not less than 6 square meters for one pharmacist working therein with additional 2 square meters for each additional pharmacist.

   c)   The height of the premises shall be at least 2.5 meters.

   d)   The floor of the pharmacy shall be smooth and washable.

   e)   The walls shall be plastered or tiled or oil painted so as to maintain smooth, durable and washable surface devoid of holes, cracks and crevices.

   f)   A pharmacy shall be provided with ample supply of good quality water.

   g)   The dispensing department shall be separated by a barrier to prevent the admission of the public.

3. *Furniture and apparatus:*

   a)   The furniture and apparatus of a pharmacy shall be

adapted to the uses for which they are intended and correspond to the size and requirements of the establishment. Drugs, chemicals, and medicaments shall be kept in a room appropriate to their properties and in such special containers as will prevent any deterioration of the contents or of contents of containers kept near them. Drawers, glasses and other containers used for keeping medicaments shall be of suitable size and capable of being closed tightly to prevent the entry of dust.

b)   Every container shall bear a label of appropriate size, easily readable with names of medicaments as given in the Pharmacopoeias.

c)   A pharmacy shall be provided with a dispensing bench, the top of which shall be covered with washable and impervious material like stainless steel, laminated or plastic, etc.

d)   A pharmacy shall be provided with a cupboard with lock and key for the storage of poisons and shall be clearly marked with the work 'poison' in red letters on a white background.

e)   Containers of all concentrated solution shall bear special label or marked with the works "To be diluted".

f)   A Pharmacy shall be provided with the following minimum apparatus and books necessary for making of official preparations and prescriptions:-

Apparatus: -

a)   Balance, dispensing, sensitivity 30 mg.

b)   Balance, counter, capacity 3 Kg, sensitivity 1 gm.

c)   Beakers, lipped, assorted sizes

d)   Bottles, prescription, ungraduated assorted sizes

e)   Corks assorted sizes and tapers.

f)   Cork, extracter

g)   Evaporating dishes, porcelain.

h) Filter paper

i) Funnels, glass

j) Litmus paper, blue and red

k) Measure glasses cylindrical 10 ml, 25 ml, 100 ml and 500 ml

l) Mortars and pestles, glass

m) Mortars and pestles, Wedgwood.

n) Ointment pots with Bakelite or suitable caps.

o) Ointment slab, porcelain

p) Pipettes, graduated, 2 ml, 5 ml and 10 ml

q) Ring, stand (retort) iron, complete with rings.

r) Rubber stamps and pad

s) Scissors

t) Spatulas, rubber or vulcanite

u) Spatulas, stainless steel.

v) Spirit lamp

w) Glass stirring rods

x) Thermometer, $0{}^{o}C$ to $200{}^{o}C$

y) Tripod stand

z) Watch glasses

aa) Water bath

bb) Water distillation still in case Eye drops and Eye lotions are prepared.

cc) Weights, Metric, 1 mg. to 100 gm

dd) Wire Gauze

ee) Pill finisher, boxwood

ff) Pill Machine

gg) Pill Boxes

hh) Suppository mould

Books:

a) The Indian Pharmacopoeia (current Edition)

b) National Formulary of Indian (Current Edition)

c) The drugs and Cosmetics Act, 1940

d) The Drugs and Cosmetics Rules, 1945

e) The Pharmacy Act, 1948

f) The Dangerous Drugs Act, 1930

General provisions:

a) A pharmacy shall be conducted under the continuous personal supervision of a Registered Pharmacist whose name shall be displayed conspicuously in the premises.

b) The Pharmacist shall always put on clean white overalls. The premises and fittings of the pharmacy shall be properly kept and everything shall be in good order and clean.

c) All records and registers shall be maintained in accordance with the laws in force.

d) Any container taken from the poison cupboard shall be replaced therein immediately after use and the cupboard locked. The keys of the poison cupboard shall be kept in the personal custody of the responsible person.

e) Medicaments when supplied shall have labels conforming to the provisions of laws in force.

3.11 SCHEDULE M

(*Good Manufacturing Practices and Requirements of Premises, Plant and Equipment for Pharmaceutical products.*)

I. GOOD MANUFACTURING PRACTICES FOR PREMISES AND MATERIALS

GENERAL REQUIREMENTS

1. *Location and surroundings:* The factory building(s) for manufacture of drugs shall be so situated and shall have such measures as to avoid risk of contamination from external environmental including open sewage, drain, public lavatory or any factory which product disagreeable or obnoxious odour, fumes, excessive soot, dust, smoke, chemical or biological emissions.

2. *Building and premises:* The building(s) used for the factory shall be designed, constructed, adapted and maintained to suit the manufacturing operations so as to permit production of drugs under hygienic conditions. They shall conform to the conditions laid down in the Factories Act, 1948 (63 of 1948)

   The premises used for manufacturing, processing, warehousing, packaging labelling and testing purposes shall be –

   i. Compatible with other drug manufacturing operations that may be carried out in the same or adjacent area / section;

   ii. Adequately provided with working space to allow orderly and logical placement of equipment, materials and movement of personnel so as to:

   a) Avoid the risk of mix-up between different categories of drugs or with raw materials, intermediates and in-process material;

   b) Avoid the possibilities of contamination and cross-contamination by providing suitable mechanism;

   iii. Designed / constructed / maintained to prevent entry of insects, pests, birds, vermin, and rodents. Interior surface (walls, floors and ceilings) shall be smooth and free from cracks, and permit easy cleaning, painting and disinfection;

iv. Air-conditioned, where prescribed for the operations and dosage forms under production. The production and dispensing areas shall be well lighted, effectively ventilated, with air control facilities and may have proper Air Handling Units (wherever applicable) to maintain conditions including temperature and, wherever necessary, humidity, as defined for the relevant product. These conditions shall be appropriate to the category of drugs and nature of the operation. These shall also be suitable to the comforts of the personnel working with protective clothing, products handled, and operations undertaken within them in relation to the external environment. These areas shall be regularly monitored for compliance with required specifications;

v. Provided with drainage system, as specified for the various categories of products, which shall be of adequate size and so designed as to prevent back flow and/or prevent insets and rodents entering the premises. Open channels shall be avoided in manufacturing areas and, where provided, these shall be shallow to facilitate cleaning and disinfection;

vi. The walls and floors of the areas where manufacture of drugs is carried out shall be free from cracks and open joints to avoid accumulation of dust. These shall be smooth, washable, covered and shall permit easy and effective cleaning and disinfection. The interior surfaces shall not shed particles. A periodical record of cleaning and painting of the premises shall be maintained.

3. *Water Supply:* There shall be validated system for treatment of water drawn from own or any other source to render it potable in accordance with standards specified by the Bureau of Indian Standards or Local Municipality, as the case may be, so as to produce Purified Water conforming to Pharmacopoeial specification. Purified Water so produced shall only be used for all operations except washing and cleaning operations where potable water may be used. Water shall be stored in tanks, which do not adversely affect quality of water and ensure freedom from

microbiological growth. The tank shall be cleaned periodically and records maintained by the licensee in this behalf.

4. *Disposal of waste*

i.   The disposal of sewage and effluents (solid, liquid and gas) from the manufactory shall be in conformity with the requirements of Environment Pollution Control Board.

ii.   All bio-medical waste shall be destroyed as per the provisions of the Bio-Medical Waste (Management and Handling) Rules, 1996.

iii.   Additional precautions shall be taken for the storage and disposal of rejected drugs. Records shall be maintained for all disposal of waste.

iv.   Provisions shall be made for the proper and safe storage of waste materials awaiting disposal. Hazardous, toxic substances and flammable materials shall be stored in suitably designed and segregated, enclosed areas in conformity with Central and State Legislations.

5. *Warehousing Area*

a)   Adequate areas shall be designed to allow sufficient and orderly warehousing of various categories of materials and products like starting and packaging materials, intermediates, bulk and finished products, products in quarantine, released, rejected, returned or recalled, machine and equipment spare parts and change items.

b)   Warehousing areas shall be designed and adapted to ensure good storage conditions. They shall be clean, dry and maintained with acceptable temperature limits, where special storage conditions are required (e.g. temperature, humidity), these shall be provided, monitored and recorded. Storage areas shall have appropriate house-keeping and rodent, pests and vermin control procedures and records maintained. Proper racks, bins and platforms shall be provided for the storage of materials.

c)   Receiving and dispatch bays shall protect materials and products from adverse weather conditions.

d)   Where quarantine status is ensured by warehousing in separate earmarked areas in the same warehouse or store, these areas shall be clearly demarcated. Any system replacing the physical quarantine, shall give equivalent assurance of segregation. Access to these areas shall be restricted to authorized persons.

e)   There shall be a separate sampling area in the warehousing area for active raw materials and excipients. If sampling is performed in any other area, it shall be conducted in such a way as to prevent contamination, cross-contamination and mix-up.

f)   Segregation shall be provided for the storage of rejected, recalled or returned materials or products. Such areas, materials or products shall be suitably marked and secured. Access to these areas and materials shall be restricted.

g)   Highly hazardous, poisonous and explosive materials such as narcotics, psychotropic drugs and substances presenting potential risks of abuse, fire or explosion shall be stored in safe and secure areas. Adequate fire protection measures shall be provided in conformity with the rules of the concerned civic authority.

h)   Printed packaging materials shall be stored in safe, separate and secure areas.

i)   Separate dispensing areas for ß (Beta) lactum, Sex Hormones and Cytotoxic substances or any such special categories of product shall be provided with proper supply of filtered air and suitable measures for dust control to avoid contamination. Such areas shall be under differential pressure.

j)   Sampling and dispensing of sterile materials shall be conducted under aseptic conditions conforming to Grade A, which can also be performed in a dedicated area within the manufacturing facility.

k)   Regular checks shall be made to ensure adequate steps are taken against spillage, breakage and leakage of containers.

l)   Rodent treatments (Pest control) should be done regularly and at least once in a year and record maintained.

6. Production area

a)   The production area shall be designed to allow the production preferably in uni-flow and with logical sequence of operations.

b)   In order to avoid the risk of cross-contamination, separate dedicated and self contained facilities shall be made available for the production of sensitive pharmaceutical products like penicillin or biological preparations with live micro-organisms. Separate dedicated facilities shall be provided for the manufacture of contamination causing and potent products such as Beta-Lactum, sex hormones and cytotoxic substances.

c)   Working and in-process space shall be adequate to permit orderly and logical positioning of equipment and materials and movement of personnel to avoid cross contamination and to minimize risk of omission or wrong application of any manufacturing and control measures.

d)   Pipe-work, electrical fittings, ventilation openings and similar services lines shall be designed, fixed and constructed to avoid creation of recesses. Services lines shall preferably be identified by colours and the nature of the supply and direction of the flow shall be marked/indicated.

7. Ancillary Areas

a)   Rest and refreshment rooms shall be separate from other areas. These areas shall not lead directly to the manufacturing and storage areas.

b)   Facilities for changing, storing clothes and for washing and toilet purposes shall be easily accessible and adequate for the number of users. Toilets, separate for males and females, shall not be directly connected with production or storage areas. There shall be written instructions for cleaning and disinfection of such areas.

c)   Maintenance workshops shall be separate and away from production areas. Whenever spares, changed parts and tools are stored in the production area, these shall be kept in dedicated rooms or lockers. Tools and spare parts for use in sterile areas shall be disinfected before these are carried inside the production areas.

d)   Areas housing animals shall be isolated from other areas. The other requirements regarding animal houses shall be those as prescribed in Rule 150-C(3) of the Drugs and Cosmetics Rules, 1945 which shall be adopted for production purposes.

8.   *Quality Control Area*

a)   Quality Control Laboratories shall be independent of the production areas. Separate areas shall be provided each for physico-chemical, biological, microbiological or radioisotope analysis. Separate instrument room with adequate area shall be provided for sensitive and sophisticated instruments employed for analysis.

b)   Quality Control Laboratories shall be designed appropriately for the operations to be carried out in them. Adequate space shall be provided to avoid mix-ups and cross-contamination. Sufficient and suitable storage space shall be provided for test samples, retained samples, reference standards, reagents and records.

c)   The design of the laboratory shall take into account the suitability of construction materials and ventilation. Separate air handling units and other requirements shall be provided for biological, microbiological and radioisotopes testing areas. The laboratory shall be provided with regular supply of water of appropriate quality for cleaning and testing purpose.

d)   Quality Control Laboratory shall be divided into separate sections i.e. for chemical, microbiological and wherever required, biological testing. These shall have adequate area for basis installation and for ancillary purposes. The microbiology section shall have arrangements such as airlocks and laminar air flow work station, wherever considered necessary.

9.   *Personnel*

a)   The manufacture shall be conducted under the direct supervision of competent technical staff with prescribed qualifications and practical experience in the relevant dosage and / or active pharmaceutical products.

b)   The head of the Quality Control Laboratory shall be independent of the manufacturing unit. The testing shall be conducted under the direct supervision of competent technical staff who shall be whole time employees of the licensee.

c)   Personnel for Quality Assurance and Quality Control operations shall be suitably qualified and experienced.

d)   Written duties of technical and Quality Control personnel shall be laid and following strictly.

e)   Number of personnel employed shall be adequate and in direct proportion to the workload.

f)   The licensee shall ensure in accordance with a written instruction that all personnel in production area or into Quality Control Laboratories shall receive training appropriate to the duties and responsibility assigned to them. They shall be provided with regular in-service training.

10. *Health, clothing and sanitation of workers*

a)   The personnel handling Beta-lactum antibiotics shall be tested for Penicillin sensitivity before employment and those handling sex hormones, cytotoxic substances and other potent drugs shall be periodically examined for adverse effects. These personnel should be moved out of these sections (except in dedicated facilities), by rotation, as a health safeguard.

b)   Prior to employment, all personnel, shall undergo medical examination including eye examination, and shall be free from Tuberculosis, skin and other communicable or contagious diseases. Thereafter, they should be medically examined periodically, at least once a year. Records shall be maintained thereof. The licensee shall provide the services of a qualified physician for assessing the health status of personnel involved in different activities.

c)   All persons prior to and during employment shall be trained in practices which ensure personnel hygiene. A high level of personal hygiene shall be observed by all those engaged in the manufacturing processes. Instructions to this effect shall be displayed in change rooms and other strategic locations.

d) No person showing, at any time, apparent illness or open lesions which may adversely affect the quality of products, shall be allowed to handle starting materials, packing materials, in-process materials, and drug products until his condition is no longer judged to be a risk.

e) All employees shall be instructed to report about their illness or abnormal health condition to their immediate supervisor so that appropriate action can be taken.

f) Direct contact shall be avoided between the unprotected hands of personnel and raw materials, intermediate or finished, unpacked products.

g) All personnel shall wear clean body coverings appropriate to their duties. Before entry into the manufacturing area, there shall be change rooms separate for each sex with adequate facilities for personal cleanliness such as wash basin with running water, clean towels, hand dryers, soaps, disinfectants, etc. The change room shall be provided with cabinets for the storage of personal belongings of the personnel.

h) Smoking, eating, drinking, chewing or keeping plants, food, drink and personal medicines shall not be permitted in production, laboratory, storage and other areas where they might adversely influence the product quality.

11. *Raw Materials*

a) The licensee shall keep an inventory of all raw materials to be used at any stage of manufacture of drugs and maintain records as per Schedule U.

b) All incoming materials shall be quarantined immediately after receipt or processing. All materials shall be stored under appropriate conditions and in an orderly fashion to permit batch segregation and stock rotation by a 'first in/first expiry' – 'first-out principle. All incoming materials shall be checked to ensure that the consignment corresponds to the order placed.

c)   All incoming materials shall be purchased from approved sources under valid purchase vouchers. Wherever possible, raw materials should be purchased directly from the producers.

d)   Authorized staff appointed by the licensee in this behalf, which may include personnel from the Quality Control Department, shall examine each consignment on receipt and shall check each container for integrity of package and seal. Damaged containers shall be identified, recorded and segregated.

e)   If a single delivery of material is made up of different batches, each batch shall be considered as a separate batch for sampling, testing and release.

f)   Raw materials in the storage area shall be appropriately labelled. Labels shall be clearly marked with the following information:

- Designated name of the product and the internal code reference, where applicable, and analytical reference number;

- Manufacturer's name, address and batch number;

- The status of the contents (e.g. quarantine, under test, released, approved, rejected); and

- The manufacturing date, expiry date and re-test date.

g)   There shall be adequate separate areas for materials "under test", "approved" and "rejected" with arrangements and equipment to allow dry, clean and orderly placement of stored materials and products, wherever necessary, under controlled temperature and humidity.

h)   Containers from which samples have been drawn shall be identified.

i)   Only raw materials which have been released by the Quality Control Department and which are within their shelf-life shall be used. It shall be ensured that shelf life of formulation product shall not exceed with that of active raw materials used.

j)   It shall be ensured that all the containers of raw materials are placed on the raised platforms/racks and not placed directly on the floor.

12. *Equipment.*

a)   Equipment shall be located, designed, constructed, adapted and maintained to suit the operations to be carried out. The layout and design of the equipment shall aim to minimise the risk of errors and permit effective cleaning and maintenance in order to avoid cross-contamination, build-up of dust or dirt and, in general any adverse effect on the quality of products. Each equipment shall be provided with a logbook, wherever necessary.

b)   Balances and other measuring equipment of an appropriate range, accuracy and precision shall be available in the raw material stores, production and in process control operations and these shall be calibrated and checked on a scheduled basis in accordance with Standard Operating Procedures and records maintained.

c)   The parts of the production equipment that come into contact with the product shall not be reactive, additive or adsorptive to an extent that would affect the quality of the product.

d)   To avoid accidental contamination, wherever possible, non-toxic/edible grade lubricants shall be used and the equipment shall be maintained in a way that lubricants do not contaminate the products being produced.

e)   Defective equipment shall be removed from production and Quality Control areas or appropriately labelled.

13. *Documentation and Records*

Documentation is an essential part of the Quality assurance system and, as such, shall be related to all aspects Good Manufacturing Practices (GMP). Its aim is to define the specifications for all materials, method of manufacture and control, to ensure that all personnel concerned with manufacture know the information necessary to decide whether or not to release a bath of drug for sale and to provide an audit trail that shall permit investigation of the history of any suspected defective batch.

a)   Documents designed, prepared, reviewed and controlled, wherever applicable, shall comply with these rules.

b)   Documents shall be approved, signed and dated by appropriate and authorized persons.

c)   Documents shall specify the title, nature and purpose. They shall be laid out in an orderly fashion and be easy to check. Reproduced documents shall be clear and legible. Documents shall be regularly reviewed and kept up to date. Any alteration made in the entry of a document shall be signed and dated.

d)   The records shall be made or completed at the time of each operation in such a way that all significant activities concerning the manufacture of pharmaceutical products are traceable. Records and associated Standard Operating Procedures (SOP) shall be retained for at least one year after the expiry date of the finished product.

e)   Data may be recorded by electronic data processing systems or other reliable means, but Master Formulae and detailed operating procedures relating to the system in use shall also be available in a hard copy to facilitate checking of the accuracy of the records. Wherever documentation is handled by electronic data processing methods, authorized persons shall enter modify data in the computer. There shall be record of changed and deletions. Access shall be restricted by 'passwords' or other means and the result of entry of critical data shall be independently checked. Batch records electronically stored shall be protected by a suitable back-up. During the period of retention, all relevant data shall be readily available.

14. *For product containers and closures:*

a)   All containers and closures intended for use shall comply with the pharmacopoeial requirements. Suitable validated test methods, sample sizes, specifications, cleaning procedure and sterilization procedure, wherever indicated, shall be strictly followed to ensure that these are not reactive, additive, absorptive, or leach to an extent that significantly affects the quality or purity of the drug. No second hand or used containers and closures shall be used.

b) Whenever bottles are being used, the written schedule of cleaning shall be laid down and followed. Where bottles are not dried after washing, they should be rinsed with deionised water or distilled water, as the case may be.

material, intermediate and bulk products shall be available. The specifications should be authenticated.

d) *For finished products.* - Appropriate specifications for finished products shall include:

- The designated name of the product and the code reference;

- The formula or a reference to the formula and the pharmacopoeial reference;

- Directions for sampling and testing or a reference to procedures;

- A description of the dosage form and package details;

- The qualitative and quantitative requirements, with the acceptance limits for release;

- The storage conditions and precautions, where applicable, and

- The shelf-life.

e) *For preparation of containers and closures.* - The requirements mentioned in the Schedule do not include requirements of machinery, equipments and premises required for preparation *of* containers and closures for different dosage forms and categories of drugs. The suitability and adequacy of the machinery, equipment and premises shall be examined taking into consideration the requirements of each licensee in this respect.

15. *Master Formula Records:*

There shall be Master Formula records relating to all manufacturing procedures for each product and batch size to be manufactured. These shall be prepared and endorsed by the competent technical staff i.e. head of production and quality control. The master Formula shall include: -

a)   The name of the product together with product reference code relating to its specifications;

b)   The patent or proprietary name of the product along with the generic name, a description of the dosage form, strength, composition of the product and batch size;

c)   Name, quantity, and reference number of all the starting materials to be used. Mention shall be made of any substance that may 'disappear' in the courts of processing.

d)   A statement of the expected final yield with the acceptable limits, and of relevant intermediate yields, where applicable.

e)   A statement of the processing location and the principal equipment to be used.

f)   The methods, or reference to the methods, to be used for preparing the critical equipments including cleaning, assembling, calibrating, sterilizing.

g)   Detailed stepwise processing instructions and the time taken for each step;

h)   The instructions for in-process control with their limits;

i)   The requirements for storage conditions of the products, including the container, labelling and special storage conditions where applicable;

j)   Any special precautions to be observed; and

k)   Packing details and specimen labels.

16. *Batch* Processing *Records*

a)   There shall be Batch Processing Record for each product. It shall be based on the relevant parts of the currently approved Master Formula. The method of preparation of such records included in the Master Formula shall be designed to avoid transcription errors.

b)   Before any processing begins, check shall be performed and recorded to ensure that the equipment and work station are clear of previous products, documents or materials not required for the planned process are removed and the equipment is clean and suitable for use.

c)   During processing, the following information shall be recorded at the time each action is taken and the record shall be dated and signed by the person responsible for the processing operations: -

- The name of the product

- The number of the batch being manufactured,

- Dates and time of commencement, of significant intermediate stages and of completion of production,

- Initials of the operator of different significant steps of production and where appropriate, of the person who checked each of these operations,

- The batch number and/or analytical control number as well as the quantities of each starting material actually weighed,

- Any relevant processing operation or event and major equipment used,

- A record of the in-process controls and the initials of the person(s) carrying them out, and the results obtained,

- The amount of product obtained after different and critical stages of manufacture (yield),

- Comments or explanations for significant deviations from the expected yield limits shall be given.

- Notes on special problems including details, with signed authorization, for any deviation from the Master Formula.

- Addition of any recovered or reprocessed material with reference to recovery or reprocessing stages,

17. *Quality Control System:*

Quality control shall be concerned with sampling, specifications, testing, documentation, release procedures which ensure that the necessary and relevant tests are actually carried and that the materials are not released for use, nor products released for sale or supply until their quality has been judged to be satisfactory. It is not confined to laboratory operations but shall be involved n all decisions concerning the quality of the product. It shall be ensured that all quality control arrangements are effectively and reliably carried out the department as a whole shall have other duties such as to establish evaluate, validate and implement all Quality Control Procedures and methods.

a) Every manufacturing establishment shall establish its own quality control laboratory manner by qualified and experience staff.

b) The area of the quality control laboratory may be divided into Chemical, Instrumentation, Microbiological and Biological testing.

c) Adequate area having the required storage conditions shall be provided for keeping reference samples. The quality control department shall evaluate, maintain and store reference samples.

d) Standard operating procedures shall be available for sampling, inspecting and testing of raw materials, intermediate bulk finished products and packing materials and, wherever necessary, for monitoring environmental conditions.

e) There shall be authorized and dated specifications for all materials, products, reagents and solvents including test of identity, content, purity and quality. These shall include specifications for water, solvents and reagents used in analysis.

f)   No batch of the product shall be released for sale or supply until it has been certified by the authorized person(s) that it is in accordance with the requirements of the standards laid down.

g)   Reference/retained samples from each batch of the products manufactured shall be maintained in quantity which is at least twice the quantity of the drug required to conduct all the tests, except sterility and pyrogen/Bacterial Endotoxin Test performed on the active material and the product manufactured. The retained product shall be kept in its final pack or simulated pack for a period of three months after the date of expiry.

h)   Assessment of records pertaining to finished products shall include all relevant factors, including the production conditions, the results of in process testing, the manufacturing (including packaging) documentation, compliance with the specification for the finished product, and an examination of the finished pack. Assessment records should be signed by the in-charge of production and countersigned by the authorised quality control personnel before a product is released for sale or distribution.

i)   Quality control personnel shall have access to production areas for sampling and investigation, as appropriate.

j)   The quality control department shall conduct stability studies of the products to ensure and assign their shell life at the prescribed conditions of storage. All records of such studies shall be maintained.

k)   The in-charge of Quality Assurance shall investigate all product complaints and records thereof shall be maintained.

l)   All instruments shall be calibrated and testing procedures validated before these are adopted for routine testing. Periodical calibration of instrument and validation of procedures shall be carried out.

m)   Each specification for raw materials, intermediates, final products, and packing materials shall be approved and maintained by the Quality Control Department. Periodic revisions of the specifications shall be carried out wherever changes are necessary.

n)   Pharmacopoeia, reference standards, working standards, references, spectra, other reference materials and technical books, as required, shall be available in the Quality Control Laboratory of the licensee.

18. *Labels and other Printed Materials:*

Labels are absolutely necessary for identification of the drugs and their use. The Printing shall be done in bright colours and in a legible manner. The label shall carry all the prescribed details about the product.

a)   All containers and equipment shall bear appropriate labels. Different colour coded tablets shall be used to indicate the status of a product (for example under test, approved, passed, rejected).

b)   To avoid chance mix-up of printed packaging materials, product leaflets, relating to different products, shall be stored separately.

c)   Prior to release, all labels for containers, cartons and boxes and all circulars, inserts and leaflets shall be examined by the Quality Control Department of the licensee.

d)   Prior to packaging and labelling of a given batch of a drug, it shall be ensured by the licensee that samples are drawn from the bulk and duly tested, approved and released y the quality control personnel.

e)   Records of receipt of all labelling and packaging materials shall be maintained for each shipment received indicating receipt, control reference numbers and whether accepted or rejected. Unused coded and damaged labels and packaging materials shall be destroyed and recorded.

f)   The label or accompanying document of reference standards and reference culture shall indicate concentration, lot number, potency, date on which containers was first opened and storage conditions, where appropriate.

REQUIREMENTS FOR PLANT AND EQUIPMENTS

S.no	CATEGORY	AREA	EQUIPMENTS
1.	Semisolid preparations (Ointments, Emulsions, Lotions, Suspensions)	30m^2	Mixing tank.Kettle.Power driven mixes.Storage tanks.Colloidal mill.Triple roller mill.Liquid fluid equipment.Jar/tube filling equipment.
2.	Oral liquids (Syrups, Elixirs, Solutions)	30m^2	Mixing and storage tank.Portable mixer.Filter press. Vacuum or gravity filter. Water still.Pilfer proof cap sealing machine. Clarity testing table.
3.	Solid unit dosage forms (Pills, Tablets, Hypodermic tablets)	Granulating area (30m^2)	Disintegrator.Powder mixer.Mass mixer.Granulator.Ovens.
		Compression area (30m^2)	Tablet machine.Pill machine.Punch and die.Tablet counter.Tablet inspection table.Hardness tester.Weighing balance.D.T apparatus.
		Coating area (30m^2)	Jacketed kettle.Coating pan.Polishing pan.Heater and exhaust systems.Air-conditioning and dehumidification.
4.	Powders	30m^2	Disintegrators.Mixer.Sifter.S.S. vessels.Scoops.Filling equipments.
5.	Filling of hard gelatine capsule.	25m^2	Mixing and blending machines.Capsule filling units.Capsule counter.
6.	Ophthalmics (Ointments, Lotions)	25m^2	Hot air oven.Kettle.Colloidal mill.Tube filling equipments.Mixing and storage tanks.Sintered glass filters.Seitz filter.Liquid filling machines.Autoclave.

Continued from previous page

S.no	CATEGORY	AREA	EQUIPMENTS
7.	Pessaries and suppositories.	30m²	Mixing and pouringequipment.Moulding equipment.Mixer.Granulator. Drier. Compressing machine.Counter.
		Totally 60m² Manufacturing area	Storage equipment for ampoules, vials, bottles and closures. Washing and drying equipments.Dust proof storage cabinet.Water still.Mixing and preparation tank.Filter press.Autoclave.Hot air oven.
8.	Parentral preparation.	Filling and sealing area.	Benches.Filling and sealing units.
		Aseptic filling/sealing.	Bacteriological table.Filling and sealing units.
		General room.	Inspection table.Leak testing equipment.Labelling and packing benches.Finished goods storage.

3.12 SCHEDULE-Y

(Requirements and Guidelines on Clinical Trials for Import and Manufacture of New Drug.)

1.   CLINICAL TRIALS.

Nature of trials:

The clinical trials required to be carried out in the country before a new drug is approved for marketing depend on the status of the drug in other countries. If the drug is already approved/marketed, Phase III trials as required. If the drug is not approved/marketed trials are generally allowed to be initiated at one phase earlier to the phase of trials in other countries.

For new drug substances discovered in other countries phase I trials are not usually allowed to be initiated in India unless Phase I data as required are avialable. However, such trials may be permitted even in the absence of Phase I data from other countries if the drug is of special relevance to the health problem of India.

For new drug substances discovered in India, clinical trials are required to be carried out in India right from phase I as required, though Phase III as required, permission to carry out these trials is generally given in stages, considering the data emerging from earlier phase.

Permission for trials:

Permission to initiate clinical trials with a new drug may be obtained by applying in Form 12 for a test licence (TL) to import or manufacture the drug under the Rules. Data appropriate for the various phases of clinical trials to be carried out should accompany the application as per format given. In addition, the protocol for proposed trials, case report forms to be used, and the names of investigators and institutions should also be submitted for approval. The investigators selected should possess appropriate qualifications and experience and should have such investigations facilities as are germane to the proposed trials protocol.

Permission to carry out clinical trials with a new drug is issued along with a test licence in Form 11.

It is desirable that protocols for clinical trials be reviewed and approved by the institution's ethical committee. Since such committees at present do not exist in all institutions, the approval granted to a protocol by the ethical committee of one institution will be applicable to use of that protocol in other institutions which do not have an ethical committee. In case none of the trial centres/institutions has an ethical committee, the acceptance of the protocol by the investigator and its approval by the Drugs Controller (India) or any officer as authorized by him to do so will be adequate to initiate the trials.

For new drugs having potential for use in children, permission for clinical trials in the paediatric age group is normally given after phase III trials as required under item 7 of the said Appendix in adults are completed. However, if the drug is of value primarily in a disease of children, early trials in the paediatric age group may be allowed.

Responsibilities of Sponsor/Investigator:

Sponsors are required to submit to the licensing authority as given under Rule 21 an annual status report on each clinical trial, namely, ongoing, completed, or terminated. In case a trial is terminated, reason for this should be stated.

Any unusual, unexpected or serious adverse drug reaction (ADR) detected during a trial should be promptly communicated by the sponsor to the licensing authority under Rule 21 and the other investigators.

In all trials an informal, written consent required to be obtained from each volunteer/patient in the prescribed Forms which must be signed by the patient/volunteer and the chief investigator.

2.   CHEMICAL AND PHARMACEUTICAL INFORMATION:

a)   Generic name and/or any other approved name with dosage form and strength should be provided.

b)   Patent status described.

c)   Brief description about physical, chemical, biological properties of drug such as neutralizing equivalents, solubility, partition co-efficient, hygroscopicity, crystal properties, X-ray, melting point, boiling point etc.

3. ANIMAL TOXICOLOGY.

Acute Toxicology:

Acute toxicity studies (See Appendix I item 4.2) should be carried out in at least two species usually mice and rats using the same route as intended for humans. In addition, at least one more route should be used to ensure systemic absorption of the drug; this route may depend on the nature of the drug. Mortality should be looked for up to 72 hours after parentral administration and up to 7 days after oral administration. Symptoms, signs and mode of death should be reported, with appropriate macroscopic and microscopic findings where necessary. LD 50s should be reported preferably with 95 per cent confidence limited, if LD 50s cannot be determined, reasons for this should be stated.

Long term toxicity:

Long term toxicity should be carried out in at least two mammalian species, of which one should be a non rodent. The duration of study will depend on whether the application is for marketing permission or for clinical trial, and in the latter case, on the phase of trials. If a species is known to metabolize the drug in the same way as humans, it should be preferred.

In long-term toxicity studies the drug should be administered 7 days a week by the route intended for clinical use in humans. The number of animals required for these studies, i.e. the minimum number on which data should be available.

A control group of animals given the vehicle along should always be included and three other groups should be given graded dose of the drug; the highest dose should produce observable toxicity, the lowest dose should not cause observable toxicity, but should be comparable to the intended therapeutic dose in humans of a multiple of it, e.g. 2.5 to make allowance for the sensitivity of the species; the intermediate dose should cause some symptoms, but not gross toxicity or death, and may be placed logarithmically between the other two doses.

The variables to be monitored and recorded in long-term toxicity studies should include behavioural, physiological, biochemical, and microscopic observations.

Reproduction studies:

Reproduction studies need to be carried out only if the new drug is proposed to be studied or used in women or childbearing age.

Two species should generally be used, one of them being a non-rodent if possible.

a) Fertility Studies: The drug should be administered to both males and females, beginning a sufficient number of days before mating. In females the medication should be continued after mating and the pregnant one should be treated throughout pregnancy. The highest dose used should not affect general health or growth of the animals. The route of administration should be the same as for therapeutic use in humans. The control and the treated group should be similar size and large enough to give at least 20 pregnant animals in the control group of rodents and at least 8 pregnant animals in the control group of non-rodents. Observations should include total examination of the litters from both the groups, including spontaneous abortions, if any.

b) Teratogenicity studies: The drug should be administered throughout the period of organogenesis, using three dose levels. One of the doses should cause minimum maternal toxicity and one should be proposed dose for clinical use in humans or a multiple of it. The route of administration should be the same as for human therapeutic use. The control and the treated group should consist of at least 20 pregnant females in case of non-rodents, on each dose used. Observations should include the number of implantation sites; resorptions if any; and the number of foetuses with their sexes, weights and malformations, if any.

c) Perinatal studies: The drug should be administered throughout the last third of pregnancy and then through lactation of weaning. The control of each treated group should have at least 12 pregnant females and the dose which causes low foetal loss should be continued throughout lactation weaning. Animals should be sacrificed and observations should include macroscopic autopsy and where necessary, histopathology.

d) Local toxicity: These studies are required when the new drug is proposed to be used topically in humans. The drug should be applied to an appropriate site to determine local effects in a suitable species such as guinea pigs or rabbits, if the drug is absorbed from the site of applications, appropriate systemic toxicity studies will be required.

  e) *Mutagenicity and Carcinogenicity:* These studies are required to be carried out if the drug or its metabolite is related to a known carcinogen or when the nature and action of the drug is such as to suggest a carcinogenic/mutagenic potential. For carcinogenicity studies, at least two species should be used. These species should not have a high incidence of spontaneous tumors and should preferably be known to metabolize the drug in the same manner as humans. At least three dose levels should be used; the highest dose should be sublethal out cause observable toxicity; the lowest dose should be comparable to the intended human therapeutic dose or a multiple of it, e.g. 2.5 X; to make intermediate dose to be placed logarithmically between the other two doses. A control group should always be included. The drug should be administered 7 days a week or a fraction of the life span comparable to the fraction of human life span over which the drug is likely to be used therapeutically. Observations should include macroscopic changes observed at autopsy and detailed histopathology.

4. *ANIMAL PHARMACOLOGY:*

  Specific pharmacological actions are those with therapeutic potential for humans. These should be described according to the animal models and species used.

  Wherever possible, dose-response relationships and ED 50s should be given. Special studies to elucidate mode of action may also be described.

  General pharmacological action is effects on other organs and systems, especially cardiovascular, respiratory and central nervous systems.

  Pharmacokinetic data help relate drug effect to plasma concentration and should be given to the extent available.

5. *HUMAN/CLINICAL PHARMACOLOGY (PHASE I):*

  The objective of phase I of trials is to determine the maximum tolerated dose in humans; pharmacodynamic effects; adverse reactions, if any, with their nature and intensity; and pharmacokinetic behaviour of the drug as far as possible. These studies are carried out in healthy adult males, using clinical, physiological and biochemical observations. At least 2 subjects should be used on each dose.

Phase I trials are usually carried out by investigators trained in clinical pharmacology and having the necessary facilities to closely observe and monitor the subjects. These may be carried out at one or two centres.

6. EXPLANATORY TRIALS (PHASE II):

In phase II trial a limited number of patients are studies carefully to determine possible therapeutic use, effective dose range and further evaluation of safety and pharmacokinetics. Normally 10-12 patients should be studied at each dose level. These studies are usually limited to 3-4 centres and carried out by clinicians specialized in the concerned therapeutic areas and having adequate facilities to perform the necessary investigations for efficacy and safety.

7. CONFIRMATORY TRIALS (PHASE III):

The purpose of these trials is to obtain sufficient evidence about the efficacy and safety of the drug in a larger number of patients, generally in comparison with a standard drug and/or a placebo as appropriate. These trials may be carried out by clinicians in the concerned therapeutic areas, having facilities appropriate to the protocol. If the drug is already approved/marketed in other countries, phase III data should generally obtained on at least 100 patients distributed over 3-4 centres primarily to confirm the efficacy and safety of the drug, in Indian patients when used as recommended in the product monograph for the claims made.

If the drug is a new drug substance discovered in India and not marketed in any other country, phase III data should be obtained at least 500 patients distributed over 10-15 centres. In addition, data on adverse drug reactions observed during clinical use of the drug should be collected in 1000-2000 patients; such data may be collected through clinicians who give written consent to use the drug as recommended and to provide a report on its efficacy and adverse during reactions in the treated patients. The selection of clinicians for such monitoring and supply of drug to them will need approval of the licensing authority under Rule 21.

8. SPECIAL STUDIES:

a) These include studies on solid oral dosage form, such as, bio-availability and dissolution studies. These are required to be submitted on the formulations manufactured in the country.

b) These include studies to explore additional aspects of the drug, e.g. use in elderly patients or patients with renal failure, secondary or ancillary effects, interactions, etc.

9. SUBMISSION OF REPORTS:

The reports of completed clinical trials shall be submitted by the applicant duly signed by the investigator with a stipulated period of time. The applicant should do so even if he is no longer interested to market the drug in the country unless there are sufficient reasons for not doing so.

10. REGULATORY STATUS IN OTHER COUNTRIES:

It is important to state if any restrictions have been placed on the use of the drug in any other country, e.g. dosage limited, exclusion of certain age groups, warnings about adverse drug reaction, etc.

Likewise, if the drug has been withdrawn from any country especially by a regulatory directive, such information should be furnished along with reasons and their relevance, if any, to India.

11. MARKETING INFORMATION:

The product monograph should comprise the full prescribing information necessary to enable a physician to use the drug properly. It should include description, actions, indications, dosage precaution, drug interactions, warnings and adverse reactions.

The drafts of label and carton texts should comply with provisions of Rules 96 and 97 of the said rules.

12. POST-MARKETING SURVEILLANCE STUDY:

On approval of a new drug, the importer or the manufacturer shall conduct post-marketing surveillance study of that new drug after getting the protocols and the names of the investigators approved by the

Licensing Authority as defined under clause (b) of Rule 21 during the initial period of two years of marketing.

REVIEW QUESTIONS

ESSAY QUESTIONS

1. Explain Drug Technical Advisory Board and Drug consultative committee and their Function.
2. Write a note on Qualification, Duties and Procedures of Government Analyst.
3. Write a note on Qualification, Powers and Procedures of Drug Inspector.
4. Write a note on Schedule O.
5. Explain the requirements for the Labelling of medicines.
6. Explain in detail Schedule N.
7. Write a note on Schedule M.
8. Explain Schedule Y.

SHORT QUESTIONS

1. Define the following.
    a) Drug.
    b) Cosmetics.
    c) Adulterated drug.
    d) Misbranded drug.
    e) Spurious drug.
    f) New drug.
    g) Government analyst.
    h) Inspector.
    i) Patent or proprietary medicine.
2. Write a note on Central Drug Laboratory.

3. Define.

    a) Schedule G.

    b) Schedule H.

    c) Schedule M.

    d) Schedule O.

    e) Schedule J.

    f) Schedule C.

    g) Schedule X.

    h) Schedule Y.

4. What type of Drugs and Cosmetics are prohibited for the provision of Import under the D&C Act 1940?

5. What are the conditions to be fulfilled for the Import of Schedule C/C_1 and Schedule X.

6. Write a note on Import of Drugs without licence.

7. Write a note on various Offences and Penalties under the provision of Import under the D&C Act 1940.

8. Write a note on various types of Manufacturing licence along with the Application Form numbers.

9. What are the conditions to be fulfilled for the manufacturing of drugs other than those specified under Schedule C/C_1 and Schedule X.

10. What are the conditions to be fulfilled for the manufacturing of drugs specified under Schedule C/C_1?

11. What are the conditions to be fulfilled for the manufacturing of drugs specified under Schedule X.?

12. Write a note on Manufacturing under Loan Licence.

13. Write a note on Manufacturing under Repackaging Licence.

14. Explain various Offence and Penalties under the provision of Manufacturing under the D&C Act 1940.

15. Write a note on various types of Sales Licence along with their Form Numbers.

16. Write a note on sales of drugs under General Licence.

17. Write a note on sales of drugs under Restricted Licence.

18. Write a note on sales of drugs through Motor Vehicle.

19. Enlist drugs included in Schedules C/C$_1$ and Schedule X.

20. Enlist the various diseases included under Schedule J.

MCQ's

1. The Drugs and Cosmetics Act was passed in year,

    a) 1904

    b) 1914

    c) 1940

    d) 1944

2. List of drugs exempted from the provision of import is included under,

    a) Schedule A

    b) Schedule B

    c) Schedule C

    d) Schedule D

3. List of incurable diseases are included under,

    a) Schedule E

    b) Schedule J

    c) Schedule H

    d) Schedule M

4. List of drugs marketed under generic names only are included in,

    a) Schedule N

    b) Schedule W

c) Schedule X

d) Schedule Y

5. Standards for disinfectants are covered under,

a) Schedule O

b) Schedule P

c) Schedule Q

d) Schedule R

6. Which of the following class of the drug is prohibited for the provision of import?

a) Schedule C drugs.

b) Schedule X drugs.

c) Schedule J.

Xd)   None of the above.

7. Licence of import of drug is obtained on application to,

a) State government.

b) Central government.

c) Drug controller of India.

d) Drug inspector.

8. Without licence one can import ___ quantity of drug for personal use.

a) 10 average doses.

b) 100 average doses.

c) 1000 average doses.

d) None of the above.

9. The Form number in order to apply for manufacturing of schedule X drugs under own premises is,

a) 27-A

b) 27-B

c) 28-A

d) 28-B

10. One of the following is NOT a type is sales licence.

   a) Wholesale.

   b) Retail.

   c) Vendor.

   d) None of the above.

11. The Form number in order to apply for retail sales of schedule X drugs is,

   a) 19

   b) 19-C

   c) 20-F

   d) 21

12. DTAB

   a) Drugs technical advisory board.

   b) Drugs technical administration board.

   c) Drugs technical analytical board.

   d) None of the above.

13. DCC.

   a) Drugs control committee.

   b) Drugs commercial committee.

   c) Drugs consultative committee.

   d) None of the above.

14. CDL.

   a) Central drugs league.

   b) Central drugs laboratory.

c) Consultative drugs laboratory.

d) None of the above.

15. In DTAB, Director of Central Research Institute is,

a) Elected member.

b) Nominated member.

c) Ex-officio member.

d) None of the above.

Answers: 1-c, 2-d, 3-b, 4-b, 5-a, 6-c, 7-c, 8-b, 9-b, 10-d, 11-b, 12-a, 13-c, 14-b, 15-c.

Chapter 4

MEDICINAL AND TOILET PREPARATION (EXCISE DUTIES) ACT 1955

4.1 INTRODUCTION

It is an Act to provide for the levy and collection of duties of excise on medicinal and toilet preparations containing alcohol, narcotic drug or narcotic

Alcohol is used as a euphoric drink and also in medicinal and toilet preparations. Using alcohol for pleasure (drinking) is an abuse, while using it for toilet preparations is pleasure and for medicinal preparation it is a necessity. Due to these reasons the alcohol used for drinking and toilet preparations are charged with higher rates of excise duties as compared to that charged for use of alcohol in medicinal preparations.

As there are three different rate of excise duty as per the purpose, it is essential to control the issue and transport of alcohol. Previously it was governed by state governments. Each state had its own rules and rate of excise duty. This led to interstate smuggling.

To overcome this difficulty and bring about uniformity in duty throughout the country Medicinal and Toilet preparation (Excise duty) Act was passed in 1955 and then amended in 1975 and 1976.

It extends to the whole of India. It shall come into force on such date, as the Central Government may, by notification in the official Gazette, appoint.

OBJECTIVES

1.   Levy and collection of excise duties on medicinal and toilet preparations containing alcohol and other narcotic drugs.

2.   To establish uniformity of excise duties throughout the country.

DEFINITIONS

1.   *Alcohol:* Means ethyl alcohol of any strength and purity having chemical compositions C_2H_5OH.

2.   *Dutiable goods:* Means the medicinal and toilet preparations specified in the schedule as being subject to the duties of excise levied under this Act.

3.   *Medicinal preparation:* Includes all drugs which are a remedy or "prescription" prepared for internal or external use of human beings or animals and all substances intended to be used for or in the treatment, mitigation or prevention of disease in human beings or animals.

4.   *Toilet preparation:* Means any preparation which is intended for use in the toilet of the human body or in perfuming apparel of any description, or any substance intended to cleanse, improve or alter the complexion, skin, hair or teeth, and includes deodorants and perfumes.

5.   *Restricted preparations:* Means every medicinal and toilet preparation specified in schedule and preparations declared by the Central Government as restricted preparation.

6.   *Excise officer:* Means an officer of the Excise Department of any State and includes any person empowered by the collecting Government to exercise all or any of the powers of an excise officer under this Act.

7.   *Absolute alcohol:* Means alcohol conforming to british pharmacopoeial standards for dehydrated alcohol.

8. *Rectified spirit:* Means plain undenatured alcohol of strength not less than 50.0° over proof and includes absolute alcohol.

9. *Denatured alcohol (spirit):* Means alcohol of any strength which has been rendered unfit for human consumption by addition of substances approved by the Central Government or State Government.

10. *Bonded laboratories (with bond):* Means premises approved and licensed for the manufacture and storage of medicinal and toilet preparations containing alcohol, opium, Indian hemp or other narcotic drugs on which duty has not been paid.

11. *Non-bonded laboratories (without bond):* Means premises approved and licensed for the manufacture and storage of medicinal and toilet preparations containing alcohol, opium, Indian hemp or other narcotic drugs on which duty has been paid.

12. *Spirit store:* Means the portion of bonded or non-bonded laboratories which is apart for the storage of alcohol, opium, Indian hemp and other narcotic drugs.

4.2 LICENSING PROCEDURE

License is required for the manufacture of preparations containing alcohol or narcotic substances.

Procedure for obtaining licence

1. Every person desiring to engage in operations requiting the possession of a licence shall apply in writing every year for a licence or for renewal thereof to the licensing authority who shall be-

    a) The Excise Commissioner in the case of a bonded manufactory or warehouse.

    b) In other cases such officer as the State Government may authorize in this behalf.

2. If any person desires to have more than one kind of licence he shall submit a separate application for every such licence.

3. Where the applicant has more than one place of business he shall obtain separate licence in respect of each such place of business.

Form of application

1. Every application for a licence under these rules shall be in such one of the proper forms of application as may be appropriate to the case, shall clearly describe the premises, if any, in which the applicant intends to conduct his business and shall be submitted so as to reach the licensing authority at least two months before the proposed date of commencement of the working of the licence. In case of renewal such application shall be submitted at least one month the commencement of the year for which it is required.

2. Every such application for grant or renewal of licence shall, where a free is prescribed in the sub-joined table, be accompanied by a treasury *chalan* showing payment of such fee: Provided that where an application for the renewal of licence is not made within the period prescribed by sub-rule (I), it shall be accompanied by an additional fee, payable the same manner, equivalent to twenty-five percent, such fee or rupee one, whichever higher.

Details to be furnished

1. Name/address of the applicant.

2. Place/state in which bonded laboratory is proposed to be built.

3. If applicant be a firm, name/address of the partners.

4. If it be a company, its registered name/address, name/address of its Directors, Managers and Managing agents.

5. Amount of capital proposed to be invested.

6. The number and full description of vats, stills and other apparatus and machinery.

7. Maximum quantity of alcohol at any one time to remain, in the form of finished and unfinished preparation.

8. The approximate date to start the preparation.

9. Statement whether the laboratory will require a whole time or part time excise officer.

10. List of preparation stating the percentage of alcohol contained and license held under Drug and Cosmetic Act- 1940.

11. Site and elevation plan of laboratory building. If quarters for excise officer are to be provided, their plans also to be submitted.

12. In case of firm, a copy of partnership-deed and in case of company-

· List of Directors/Managers.

· Copies of Memorandum of Association.

· Article of Association.

· Latest Balance Sheet.

The table below gives the different types of license issued according to the purpose and the fees applicable for such license.

S.no	PURPOSE FOR WHICH LICENCE IS REQUIRED.	LICENCE FEE PAYABLE PER ANNUM
1.	Manufacture under bond for payment of duty- (a) Allopathic medicinal preparations and toilet preparations containing alcohol— (i) where, in the alcohol consumed, the pure alcohol content is more than 2250 litres per annum (ii) where, in the alcohol consumed, the pure alcohol content is more than 2250 litres per annum (b) Medicinal preparations and toilet preparations not containing alcohol, but containing opium, Indian hemp, or other narcotic drug or narcotic (c) Homoeopathic preparations containing alcohol- (i) where, in the alcohol consumed, the pure alcohol content is more than 2250 litres per annum	200 400 20 200

Continued on Next Page

S.no	PURPOSE FOR WHICH LICENCE IS REQUIRED.	LICENCE FEE PAYABLE PER ANNUM
	(ii) where, in the alcohol consumed, the pure alcohol content is more than 2250litres per annum	400
	(d) Medical preparations is Ayurvedic, Unani or other indigenous systems of medicines containing alcohol and which are prepared by distillation or to which alcohol has been added.	50
2.	Manufacture outside bond- (a) Allopathic medicinal preparations and toilet preparations containing alcohol-	
	(i) Where in the alcohol consumed, the pure alcohol is 70 litres or less per annum.	20
	(ii) Where, in the alcohol consumed, the pure alcohol is more than 70 litres but less than 280 litres per annum.	50
	(iii) where, in the alcohol consumed, the pure alcohol is 280 litres or more per annum	400
	(b) Medicinal preparations and toilet preparations not containing alcohol but containing opiim, Indian hemp or other narcotic drug or narcotic	20
	(c) Homoeopathic preparations containing alcohol- (i) Where, in the alcohol consumed, the pure alcohol is 70 litres or less per annum.	20
	(ii) Where, in the alcohol consumed, the pure alcohol is more than 70 litres but less than 280 litres per annum.	50
	(iii) Where, in the alcohol consumed, the pure alcohol is 280 litres or more per annum.	400
	(d) Medicinal preparations in Ayurvedic, Unani or other indigenous systems of medicines containing alcohol and which are prepared by distillation or to which alcohol has been added	50

Continued on Next Page

S.no	PURPOSE FOR WHICH LICENCE IS REQUIRED.	LICENCE FEE PAYABLE PER ANNUM
3.	Manufacture of medicinal preparations containing self generated alcohol in Ayurvedic or Unani or other indigenous systems of medicines by Ayurvedic or Unani practitioners for dispensing for the use of their patients and not for sale to general public	02
4.	Bonded warehouse.	50
5.	Manufacture of medicinal preparations containing alcohol by hospitals, dispensaries and other charitable institutions which are eligible from exemption from duty under rule 7 and which are specifically authorized in this behalf by the State Government or by the Administration in the case of a Union Territory.	NIL

Grant of a license

1. On receipt of the application, the licensing authority may make such inquiries for verification of the details stated in the application and also such other inquires as it deems necessary. If the authority is satisfied that the conditions for the grant of the licence applied for have been complied with, it shall grant the applicant an appropriate licence.

2. In fixing the quantity of alcohol while issuing the license under sub-rule (1) to any manufacturer, licensing authority shall satisfy itself about the requirements of alcohol of that manufacturer and if that authority is of the opinion, that the quantity of alcohol asked for is not in conformity with the *bona fide* needs of the manufacturer, it shall either reduce or refix the quantity of alcohol as it may deem fit.

Form of licence-Limitations

1. Every licence granted or renewed under these rules shall be in such one of the proper forms of licence as may be appropriate, shall have

reference only to the premises, if any, described in the licence, and shall be for a period not exceeding one year but in no case shall such period extend beyond 31st March, next following the date of commencement of the licence.

2.   Every licence shall be deemed to have been granted or renewed personally to the licensee and no licence shall be sold or transferred.

3.   Where a licensee sells or transfers his business to another person, the purchaser or the transferee shall obtain a fresh licence under these rules but it shall be granted free of fee for the residue of the period covered by the original licence.

4.   If the holder of a licence wishes to enter into partnership in regard to the business covered by the licence he shall do so after obtaining the previous sanction of the licensing authority and his licence shall thereafter be suitably amended. Where a partnership is entered into, the partner as well as the original holder of the licence shall be bound by the conditions of that licence.

5.   If a partnership is dissolved, every person who was a partner immediately before such dissolution shall send a report of the dissolution to the licensing authority within ten days thereof.

6.   If during the currency of a licence the licensee desires to transfer his business to new premises he shall intimate his intention to the licensing authority at least fifteen days, in advance, specifying the address of the new premises, and get his licence suitably amended. The licence shall, thereupon, hold well in respect of the new premises.

Alteration or substitution of licence

The licensing authority may, at any time call for any licence and may amend or alter it or may tender to the licensee a new licence in accordance with any further conditions which may be prescribed. No correction in the licence shall be valid unless ordered and attested by the licensing authority.

Revocation and suspension of licence

1.   Any licence granted under the rules may be revoked or suspended by the licensing authority if the holder, or any person in his employ, is

found to have committed a breach of the conditions thereof or of any of the provisions of the Act of these rules or has been convicted of an offence under Section 161, read with Sec. 139 or with Sec. 116 of the Indian Penal Code : Provided that such revocation or suspension shall be made until the holder of the licence has been given a reasonable opportunity of showing cause against the action proposed to be taken.

2. Every such order shall be in writing and shall specify the reasons for the suspension or revocation and shall be communicated to the licensee.

3. Where a licence is revoked or suspended under this rule the holder of the licence shall not be entitled to claim from the Central or State Government any compensation or refund of licence-fee for such cancellation or suspension. Which help the mind in coming to a fair conclusion of the question?

Refund of licence-fee

1. If the licence applied for is refused, the licence-fee paid, if any, with the application shall be refunded.

2. If the applicant surrenders his licence at any time either before the commencement of the licence or during the currency of the licence, he shall forfeit any claim for refund of such licence-fee in full or in proportion to the period not availed of.

Licence to be exhibited

Every licensee shall exhibit his licence (or a copy thereof, certified by the proper officer) in a conspicuous part of the licensed premises.

Regulation of business of licensee

1. The licensee shall conduct his business under the licence either personally or by an agent authorized in writing by him in this behalf.

2. The licensed premises and all the goods licensed to be dealt with shall at all times be opened to inspection by the Excise Commissioner and any other officer empowered by him in this behalf subject to the provisions of rule 58.

3. The licensee shall, when so required by the Excise Commissioner or by an officer empowered by him in this behalf, give an explanation in writing regarding any irregularity detected at his licensed premises and shall furnish any information regarding the management of the said premises. He shall answer all questions put to him to the best of his knowledge and belief. He shall also, if so required, allow any officer duly empowered by the Excise Commissioner to take samples of any of the goods he is licensed to deal in for analysis.

4. The licensee shall provide a visit-book paged and stamped by any officer empowered by the Excise Commissioner in this behalf, in which the visiting officer may record in remarks when inspecting the licensed premises. The licensee shall, on the termination of the period of the licence, deliver the visit-book, the accounts and the licence to such officer as directed by the licensing authority.

5. The licensee shall preserve invoices, each memoranda, permits and other documents relating to the consignments received and dealt with by him for a period of one year after the year to which the relate.

Additional rules especially applicable for applying for a licence to manufacture medicinal and toilet preparations in a bonded/non-bonded manufactory

In addition to the particulars required in rule 83, a person desiring to obtain a licence to establish a bonded or non-bonded manufactory shall in his application for licence furnish the following particulars-

1. The name or names, and the address or addresses of the person or persons applying; if the applicant is a firm, the name and address of every partner of the firm; and if a company, the registered name and address thereof, the names of the Directions, Managers and Managing Agents, and if there is a Managing Director, the name of such Director.

2. The amount of capital proposed to be invested in the venture.

3. The name of the place, and the site on which the building or buildings housing the bonded or non-bonded manufactory is/are situated or to be constructed.

4. The approximate date from which the applicant desires to commence working the manufactory in case the required licence is granted.

5. The number and full description of the vats, stills and other permanent apparatus and machinery which the applicant wishes to set up or work.

6. the maximum quantities in London-proof litres of alcohol and alcoholic content in unfinished and finished preparations and the maximum quantities by weight of opium, Indian hemp or other narcotic drugs and their content in unfinished and finished preparations, which are likely to remain in the manufactory at one time.

7. Whether the proposed bonded manufactory will require the service of a whole-time or part-time Excise Officer;

8. The kind and number of each licence under the Drugs and Cosmetics Act, 1940 held by the applicant; and

9. A list of all preparations which the licensee proposes to manufacture in his manufactory showing the percentage or proportion of alcohol in terms of London-proof litres contained in each such preparation containing alcohol., or of opium, Indian hemp or other narcotic drug or a narcotic, in terms of weight in preparations containing those substances, quoting the authority (pharmacopoeia) under which such preparations are proposed to be manufactured.

Plan of the manufactory to accompany the application

The applicant shall enclose with the application site and elevation plans of the manufactory building or buildings showing the location of the different rooms therein with doors and windows and also similar plans of the quarters in the case of a bonded manufactory, if the licensee is required to provide quarters for the excise staff to be posted to the bonded manufactory:

Provided that the State Government may relax the provisions of this rule in the case of *hakims* and *vaidyas* who prepare medical preparations for dispensing to their patients only and not for sale.

In case of a firm certain particulars to accompany the application

In the case of a firm of a true copy of the partnership deed and if a company, a list of the Directors and Managers, as certified by the Registrar of Joint Stock Companies, together with copies of Memorandum of Association, Articles of Association and the latest balance-sheet shall be submitted with the application.

The applicant to be in possession of the requisite licence under the Drugs and Cosmetics Act, 1940

No licence for the manufacture of medicinal and toilet preparations or renewal of such licence shall be granted to an applicant unless he holds the requisite licence under that Act for the manufacture of the said medicinal preparations.

The licence for the manufacture of medicinal and toilet preparations shall be granted only to the person who already holds a licence under the Drugs and Cosmetics Act, 1940.

Disposal of application for licence to manufacture medicinal and toilet preparation in a bonded/non-bonded manufactory by the licensing authority

(1) On receipt of an application, licensing authority shall cause such enquires to be made as it may deem necessary including enquiries into the following-

     a.   The qualifications and previous experience of technical personnel engaged in the manufacturing operation.

     b.   The equipment of the bonded and non-bonded manufactory.

     c.   Soundness of the applicant's financial position; and

     d.   Suitability of the proposed building for the establishment of manufactory.

(2) If the licensing authority is satisfied that the applicant is a fit party whom a licence for the manufacture of medicinal and toilet preparations in a bonded or nonbonded manufactory may be granted, it shall issue a licence, approve the plans submitted. If they are in order, and direct the applicant to contract or establish, as the case may be, and equip the manufactory as per approved plans. The

applicant shall modify the plans in such manner as the licensing authority may direct at any time before or after the approval of the plans. After the completion of construction and equipment of the manufactory the licensing authority shall cause a verification of the plans; the applicant then shall submit blue prints of the plans, in triplicate, for approval of the licensing authority. One copy of the same shall be retained in the office of the licensing authority; one shall be sent to the officer-in-charge or the local Excise Officer as the case may be, for record in his office and one shall be with the licensee.

Security

Before granting the licence the licensing authority shall in cases where security is required to be furnished by or under these Rules, fix the amount of such security. This security shall be furnished either in cash or in interest-bearing securities viz. Government Promissory Notes, National Savings Certificate, Post Office Savings Bank Pass-Books or Post Office Cash Certificate or in Fixed Deposit Receipts of the State Bank of India, or any other Bank duly approved by the State Government. This security is liable to be increased or decreased by the licensing authority at any time, should it consider, for any reason, that the amount so fixed is inadequate, excessive or unsuitable.

4.3 MANUFACTURING

Manufacture of medicinal and toilet preparations containing alcohol shall be permitted in bond without payment of duty as well as outside bond. In the case of manufacture in bond alcohol on which duty has not been paid shall be used under excise supervision; and in the case of manufacture outside bond, only alcohol on which duty has already been paid shall be used.

MANUFACTURE IN BOND (BONDED LABORATORIES)

REQUIREMENTS

A.   Issue of rectified spirit without payment of duty

Rectified spirit shall be issued without previous payment of duty for the manufacture of medicinal and toilet preparation door to each of its compartments. All the doors shall be secured with excise ticket locks during the absence of the officer-in-charge.

B.   Entry into and exit from a bonded manufactory

Unless otherwise ordered by the State Government there shall be only one entrance to the bonded manufactory and one door to each of its compartments. All the doors shall be secured with excise ticket locks during the absence of the officer-in-charge.

C.   Essentials of a bonded manufactory

1.   A bonded manufactory shall make provision for the following-

    a.   One plain spirit store unless the manufactory is attached to a distillery or a rectified spirit warehouse from which rectified spirit is made available as and when necessary.

    b.   At least one large room for manufacturing medicinal preparations.

    c.   One or more rooms for storing finished medicinal preparations.

    d.   Separate arrangement for manufacture of toilet preparations.

    e.   The storage of finished toilet preparations.

    f.   Accommodation with necessary furniture near the bonded premises for the officer-in-charge.

    g.   Malleable iron rods not less than 19 mm. In thickness, set not more than 102 mm. Apart, embodied in brick work up to a depth of at least 51 mm. And covered on the inside with strong wire netting or expanded metal of a mesh not exceeding 25 mm. In diameter of length in every window of the bonded premises.

    h.   A board on which the name of the room and a serial number, if any, are legibly painted in oil colour on the outside of every such room in the manufactory.

    i.   All pipes from sinks or wash-basins inside manufactory premises discharging into drains forming part of the general drainage system of the premises.

j.   All gas and electric connections with the licensed premises so fixed as to admit of the supply of gas or electricity being cut off and all the regulators or switches being securely locked at the end of the day's work.

2.   The Central Government may in special cases relax any of the provisions of Clause *(i)* To *(x)* of sub-rule (1).

D.   No additions or alterations to be made without orders

No addition or alteration shall be made in the bonded premises or in respect of the permanent fixtures therein without the previous orders of the Excise Commissioner. Plans, in triplicate showing each addition or alteration shall be submitted with the application for the necessary permission and copies disposed of in the same manner as copies of the original plans of the bonded manufactory as provided in rule 95.

E.   Arrangement of receptacles in a bonded manufactory

1.   The permanent vessels for the storage of alcohol, opium Indian, hemp and other narcotic drugs and narcotic s received under bond and all the finished preparation on which duty has not been paid shall be secured with excise ticket locks.

2.   All vessels intended to hold alcohol and liquid preparations shall be gauged by the officer-in-charge. They shall each bear a distinctive serial number and their full capacities distinctly and indelibly marked on them. A record of these details shall be kept in Form R.G. I.

3.   Table shall be computed to show contents at an inch and tenth of an inch of the depth of each such vessel.

4.4 PROCEDURE OF MANUFACTURE

Indent for rectified spirit

Rectified spirit required for manufacturing medicinal and toilet preparations shall be obtained on an indent in Form I.D.-1 countersigned by the officer-in-charge, from any distillery or spirit warehouse approved by the Excise Commissioner, the original being sent by the licensee of the bonded manufactory to the distiller the duplicate sent through the officer-in-charge to the distillery or spirit warehouse officer and the triplicate retained as office copy. The cost price of such rectified spirit shall be paid by the licensee of the bonded manufactory to the distiller. If the distillery or warehouse officer has received from the officer-in-charge of the bonded manufactory the duplicate of the indent, be shall issue the spirit required under bond, under the appropriate permit in the Form in vogue in the State for transport of rectified spirit and send the advice portion of such permit to the officer-in-charge.

Verification of rectified spirit received

Consignments of rectified spirit received under bond shall be verified in volume and strength and the receipt of such supply shall be entered in register in Form R.G.-2. Subject to the provision of rule 19 duty at the rate levied by the State Government on alcoholic liquors on all wastages shall be paid by the licensee of the bonded manufactory into a Government treasury on receipt of a demand from the officer-in-charge and a copy of the treasury receipt shall be sent to the distillery officer who shall thereupon make the necessary adjustment in his register.

Storage of rectified spirit

1. After the rectified spirit received has been verified, it shall be stored in one or more vessels in the spirit store.

2. If, in any particular case, it is proved to the satisfaction of the Excise Commissioner that the loss is *bona fide* and not due to negligence or connivance on the part of the manufacture, the duty payable in respect of such loss may be waived in full or in part according to the merits of the case.

Issues of rectified spirit from the spirit store

1. Rectified spirit shall be issued from the spirit store to the laboratory of the manufactory on a requisition of the licensee, which shall be made in Form R.Q-1, but only in such quantities as are in conformity with the formulae laid down in the relevant pharmacopoeia or the formula of the patent and proprietary medicines displayed on the label of the container in the manner prescribed in the Drugs Rules, 1945, for the time being in force, for the particular preparation for

which the alcohol is required. In the case of medicinal preparation manufactured from concentrated tinctures the exact quantity of spirit to be added to them shall be calculated after ascertaining the proof-spirit content of the concentrated tinctures by analysis by the Chemical Examiner. For this purpose two samples of not less than 142 ml. each shall be taken from each concentrated tincture, one of which shall be sent to the said Chemical Examiner for ascertaining the proof-spirit content while the other shall be retained by the officer-in-charge of the bonded manufactory until the result of analysis is known, after which it may be added to the concentrated tincture from which it was originally taken. All rectified spirit so issued shall, in the presence of the officer-in charge, be added without delay to the other materials for the preparation specified in the application. Rectified spirit shall not be issued for any purpose other than the manufacture of medicinal and toilet preparations in the laboratory.

2. Finished medicinal or toilet preparations may be transferred from the finished store to the laboratory of the manufactory, for addition to raw materials for the preparation of the same or any other kind of preparation on written requisition from the licensee. Such transfers shall be shown in the respective registers maintained and the alcohol contents shall be adjusted correctly.

Manufactured dutiable goods

Each preparation manufactured shall be registered and shall bear a distinctive serial number, which shall be known as its batch number in the register in Form R.G.-3. This Register shall also show the receipt and disposal of all alcohol issued to the laboratory from the spirit store and the quantity of finished medicinal preparation manufactured therefrom. As soon a preparation is manufactured, it shall be removed to the finished store where, after it has been carefully measured, it shall be stored in vessels provided for the purpose and accounted for in the register in Form R.G.-4. The issue of opium, Indian hemp, narcotic drugs and other narcotics shall be made under the appropriate permit and the advice portion of such permit shall be sent to the officer-in-charge.

Manufacturing vessels to bear labels

Every time the percolator, or other vessel intended for alcohol is charged there shall be attached to it a label showing the following particulars-

* ·The name and batch number of the preparation.

* The description and quantity of alcohol placed in it from time to time; and

* The date of removal of the preparation and the quantity of such preparation removed.

Sample to be taken

1. On completion of production of a medicinal or toilet preparation, the officer-in-charge shall permit the licensee to take free sample of 227 ml. on such quantity of the preparation as the officer-in-charge considers necessary for analysis in his own laboratory and declaration of the strength of alcohol and medicaments.

2. Any quantity left over after analysis shall be destroyed by the licensee in his laboratory in the presence of the officer-in-charge of the laboratory.

3. A separate account of the quantity used by the licensee for analysis shall be maintained.

4. The alcoholic strength of a preparation as declared by the licensee shall be entered by the licensee in the register in Form R.G.-3.

5. Immediately after declaration by the licensee of the alcoholic strength of a finished preparation and before such preparation is removed to the store, the licensee shall make proper entries in the register in Form R.G.-3.

6. The officer-in-charge shall check the entries and if they are found in order, he shall check the contents of as many as he thinks necessary of the vessels in which the preparation is being stored. He shall then initial on the relevant entries of the Register in Form R.G.-3 and take two samples from each batch of such finished preparation for analysis and report by the Chemical Examiner.

7. One set of samples shall be sent at once to such Chemical Examiner and a note to the effect shall be made in the register in Form R.G.-3. The report of the Chemical Examiner, when received, shall be shown to the licensee.

8. The duplicate sample of a preparation which is intended exclusively for replacement of the original sample or repetition of its analysis, when necessary, shall be kept under excise ticket lock, and shall be returned to the finished store immediately on receipt of the report of the Chemical Examiner.

9. All such samples sent shall be sealed by the officer-in-charge and the licensee of the manufactory.

10. The duplicate sample shall not be returned to the finished store in any case where –

   a) The alcohol strength of a preparation from which the sample was taken, is declared by the Chemical Examiner to be beyond the margin of 3% unless the Excise Commissioner permit standardization of such sub-standard preparation; and

   b) The preparation is declared to be a spurious preparation under these rules.

11. All samples required for analysis under these rules shall be supplied free of cost by the licensee and all expenses in connection with packing and dispatch of the samples shall be borne by him. Sample of medicinal or toilet preparation may also be taken at any time by the officer-in-charge or other superior officer and such samples shall be sent to the Chemical Examiner for analysis and check.

Storage of finished products

1. Medicinal and toilet preparation shall on completion of production be stored in bulk in jars or bottles each containing not less than 2,273 ml.

2. Such preparations ready for issue may be filled in bottles or containers of not less than 56 ml. Content.

Provided that the Excise Commissioner may be an order in writing specify that any such preparation may be filled in bottles or containers of smaller capacity.

3. Every container of a finished preparation shall bear a label showing the name of the preparation, its batch number, its alcoholic strength and the name of the manufacturer.

4. The label of each container of a preparation stored in bulk shall, in addition, indicate the actual contents in litres, its alcoholic strength and the date of storage.

5. The containers shall be kept so arranged in suitable racks as to allow ready identification of each batch.

6. Any goods stored may be left in the store room for a period of three years or for such extended period as the Excise Commissioner may, in each case, allow. The owner of the bonded laboratory shall, before the expiry of the period of three years or the extended period, if any, clear the same for consumption in the State on payment of excise duty or for removal in bond to bonded warehouse or for exportation.

Deficiency noticed in the finished store

1. A record shall be kept of all deficiencies in bulk content of any finished medicinal or toilet preparation in store by the officer-in-charge in Form R.G.-4, and a report of all such deficiencies, shall be submitted by him at the end of each quarter to the Excise Commissioner.

2. All such loss in the absence of a satisfactory explanation from the licensee shall be subject to levy of duty on the quantity so lost at penal rates which shall not be more than double the rates prescribed.

Disposal of sub-standard preparations

1. A finished medicinal or toilet preparation which is or is suspected to have deteriorated in quality may, if the manufacturer so desires, be destroyed with the permission of the Excise Commissioner in the presence of the officer-in-charge and relevant entries made in the register in Form R.G.-4.

2. The Excise Commissioner may, on an application made to him by the manufacturer, allow him to re-process a sub-standard preparation.

3. Excise duty shall not be levied on the preparation so destroyed provided the Excise Commissioner is satisfied that the deterioration of the preparation, or in the alternative its improper manufacture, was due to reasons beyond the control of the licensee.

Disposal of recovered alcohol

1. Alcohol recovered in the course of production of a medicinal or toilet preparation or distilled separately from the mark of such preparation may be used for subsequent production of the same preparation provided such alcohol is collected separately and accounted for separately.

2. In cases where the alcohol recovered from a preparation liable to duty at the lower rate is sought to be used in the manufacture of a preparation subject to higher rate of duty the duty on the preparation so manufactured shall be collected or made leviable on determination of the spirit strength of the preparation.

3. An account of recovered alcohol in a recovered alcohol vat shall be maintained by the officer-in-charge in Form R.G.-2.

4. Recovered alcohol declared by the licensee to be unfit for use shall be destroyed by him in the presence of the officer-in-charge on submission of written application. No rebate of duty shall be allowed on recovered alcohol so destroyed.

Wastage in manufacture

1. The State Government may, from time to time fix the percentage of wastage in the production of a particular medicinal or toilet preparation. Any wastage that exceeds the allowable limit and is not properly accounted for shall be charged with the duty together with such penalty not exceeding the duty leviable thereon as the Excise Commissioner may deem fit. If the alcohol in strength of a preparation is found by the Chemical Examiner to exceed the highest allowable limit by more than 3 proof degrees or to be below the lowest allowable limit, its issue from the bonded manufactory shall be withheld.

2. The licensee may be allowed to adjust the alcoholic strength or the medicaments or the ingredients of such a batch of preparation in a

suitable manner with the previous approval of the Excise Commissioner provided the process employed does not impair the therapeutic or toilet properties of the preparation in any way.

3. A sample of the preparation shall be sent to the Chemical Examiner for analysis after adjusting the spirit or medicaments or other ingredients, and issue of the adjusted batch of such preparation shall be allowed only when the Chemical Examiner's report has been found to be satisfactory.

4. When an excess of more than 20 proof degrees over the strength declared by the licensee of any batch of preparation is found by the Chemical Examiner, the true strength, as ascertained by the Chemical Examiner, shall be entered in the batch account in Form R.G.-3, and the reason for this alteration shall be briefly noted in the remarks column, and the excess duty due from the licensee or any quantity issued from the batch on payment of such duty to the credit of the Central Government (in the case of Union territories) or the State Government prior to the receipt of the Chemical Examiner's report, shall be realized by the officer-in-charge with the previous sanction of the Excise Commissioner.

5. No refund or abatement of excess duty shall be allowed on any quantity of a batch of preparation issued on payment of such duty and prior to the receipt of the Chemical Examiner's report, if the strength is found to be lower than the declared by the licensee.

Remission of duty in case of loss due to accident

In case of any accidental loss of alcohol in a bonded manufactory, otherwise than by theft, the officer-in charge shall institute necessary enquiries without delay to ascertain the cause of such loss. If such loss is found to be beyond the control of the licensee the duty on the alcohol so lost shall be remitted with the approval of the Excise Commissioner or may Exercise

Office subordinate to, the Excise Commissioner specially empowered by him.in this behalf.

Issue from a bonded manufactory

1. Issues of alcoholic preparations and preparations containing opium, Indian hemp or other narcotic drugs and narcotics shall be made from a bonded manufactory on payment of duty. The licensee shall present before the officer-in-charge an application in Form A. R-2 signed by him or by his authorized representative. The officer-in-charge shall, after checking the entries and realizing the duty payable, allow the required quantities to be removed after issuing a permit.

Provided that issues to another bonded warehouse shall be made without payment of duty under proper security governed by the rules.

2. If the licensee is also an account-holder as provided for in rule 9, duty leviable on alcohol preparations and preparations containing opium, Indian hemp or other narcotic drugs and narcotics to be issued from a bonded manufactory shall be debited in the account-current before the preparations are removed from the bonded premises.

3. Dutiable goods cannot be delivered from a bonded laboratory or bonded warehouse before 6 am and after 6 pm nor in holidays.

4. Exemptions

    a) No duty is charged if-

    ➢ Issued to bonded warehouse.

    ➢ Export outside India.

    ➢ Institutions authorised to receive duty free preparations.

    b) Manufacturer may deposit an advance sum to the credit of the collecting government and every time goods are issued and corresponding duty shall be debited.

4.5 MANUFACTURE OUTSIDE BOND (NON BONDED LABORATORIES)

REQUIREMENTS

A.   Opening and closing hours

The work of manufacture and sale in the non-bonded manufactory shall be conducted between the hours of sunrise and sunset and on such days and hours as may be fixed by the Excise Commissioner. The premises shall remain closed from the hours of sunset to sunrise each day.

B.   Building arrangements

Arrangement of the building shall be as under,

1. The portion of the non-bonded manufactory used as "laboratory" shall be separate from that used for other purpose.

2. The windows of the "spirit store", "laboratory" and "finished store" shall be fitted with malleable iron bars not less than 19 mm. in thickness, set not more than 102 mm. apart and fixed in the brick-work to a depth of at least 51 mm. at each end on the inside of each window there shall be securely fastened to the bars stout wire-netting the aperture of which shall not exceed 25 mm. In diameter.

3. There shall be only one entrance to the non-bonded manufactory and one door each to the "laboratory", "spirit", "store", and "finished store".

4. All pipes from sinks and wash-basins inside the manufactory premises shall discharge into closed drains forming part of the general drainage system of the premises.

5. All electric and gas connections with the licensed premises shall be so fixed as to admit of the supply of electricity or gas being cut off and the regulators or switch being securely locked out at the end of day's work.

6. There shall be separate "spirit store" for the rectified spirit purchased at the duty of Rs. 1.10 paise, Rs. 3.85 paise and Rs. 15.50 paise per London Proof Litre.

7. There shall be separate finished stores for medicinal and toilet preparations falling under each item of the Schedule to the Act.

8. All alterations in arrangement of building and plants shall be made only with the previous sanction of the Excise Commissioner.

9. The State Government may relax all or any of the provisions of Clause (i) to (viiii) in the case of small manufacturers whose annual consumption of alcohol does not exceed 500 litres and also in the case of those who prepare medicinal preparation for dispensing to their patients only and not for sale.

C. Receptacles

1. The permanent vessels for the storage of alcohol and finished preparations containing a alcohol in the non-bounded manufactory shall be gauged accurately and tables shall be computed to show the contents of every 20 mm. and 2 mm. of its depth.

2. The receptacles for the storage of finished preparations in the finished store shall be of metal, porcelain or glass as may be convenient and necessary.

3. Each permanent vessel shall bear a distinctive serial number, its full capacity, and the purpose for which it is to be used, distinctly and indelibly marked on it. A record of these details shall be kept in the register in the Form R.G.-1.

4. All receptacles containing alcohol, tinctures, liquid extracts or other alcoholic medicinal or toilet preparations, in the laboratory shall have affixed to them labels signed by the manufacturer or his authorized representative showing the batch number, the name of the preparations and the quantity of alcohol added in the receptacles during the course of manufacture.

5. Labels placed on macerators and percolators or carboys shall show the quantity of proof-spirit contained in them on each occasion and shall be destroyed when they are emptied and cleaned.

6. Labels on bottles filled for removal shall show among other details, which the manufacturer may require, the alcoholic contents in proof-strength and average percentage of absolute alcohol it contains.

Procedure of manufacture

Indent for rectified spirit-duty paid

1. Rectified spirit required for manufacturing medicinal and toilet preparations shall be obtained on an indent prepared in triplicate, Form I.D.-1, from any distillery or spirit warehouse approved by the Excise Commissioner, the original being sent by the licensee of the manufactory to the distiller or spirit warehouse-keeper, the duplicate to the officer-in-charge of the distillery or spirit warehouse through the proper officer and the triplicate retained by the licensee as office copy. The cost of such rectified spirit shall be paid by the licensee of the manufactory to the distiller or spirit warehouse-keeper. The licensee shall credit the duty payable on the spirit indented for into a Government treasury of the collecting

    Government and enclose the *chalan* in token of such payment, to the duplicate copy of the indent. The treasury officer shall send an advice of such payment to the officer-incharge of the distillery or spirit warehouse. The officer-in-charge of the distillery or spirit warehouse, after satisfying himself that the correct amount of duty has been paid, as evidenced by the *chalan* enclosed by the licensee and the advice of such payment received, from the treasury officer, shall order the issue of rectified spirit required. The rectified spirit shall be brought from the distillery or spirit warehouse to the manufactory covered by a permit issued by the officer-in-charge of the distillery or spirit warehouse. All such permits shall be filed along with respective indents. The rectified spirit so brought into the non-bonded manufactory shall be immediately transferred to the spirit store and the necessary accounts written up then and there in the register in Form R.G.-2. Accounts of all transactions in respect of rectified spirit purchased paying the duty of Rs. 1.10 paise, Rs. 3.85 paise and Rs. 15.50 paise per London Proof Litre shall be maintained separately.

2. Where the manufactory as well as the warehouse from which rectified spirit is to be obtained is located within the same State, the licensee may authorize the owner of the distillery or warehouse to pay the duty on his behalf before the issue of rectified spirit. On

such authorization the owner of the distillery or warehouse shall pay the amount of duty into a Government treasury to the credit of the collecting Government or in such manner as may be prescribed by the Excise Commissioner.

Restrictions on manufacture

1. The manufacturer shall not sell or transfer the rectified spirit obtained by him to any other person.

2. Medicinal preparations, containing alcohol, which are capable of being consumed as ordinary alcoholic beverages falling under item No. 1 *(ii) (c)* of the Schedule to the Act shall not be manufactured from rectified spirit on which only the duty of Rs. 1.10 paise per London Proof Litre has been paid and such preparations shall be manufactured only from rectified spirit on which a duty of Rs. 3.85 paise per London Profit Litre has been paid and the rectified spirit obtained after payment of the aforesaid duty of Rs. 3.85 paise shall be accounted for separately. (2-A) Medicinal preparations containing alcohol which are capable of being consumer as ordinary alcoholic beverages falling under either item No. 1 *(ii)(b)* or item No. 2*(iii)* of the Schedule to the Act shall not be manufactured from rectified spirit on which only the duty of Rs. 1.10 paise or Rs. 3.85 paise per London Proof Litre has been paid and such preparations shall be manufactured only from rectified spirit on which duty of Rs. 15.50 paise per London Proof Litre has been paid and the rectified spirit obtained after payment of the aforesaid duty of Rs. 15.50 paise shall be accounted for separately.

3. In no case shall the quantity of rectified spirit in the possession of the manufacturer exceed the limit fixed by the licensing authority.

Manufacture, storage and sale

1. The manufacture and storage of all preparations shall be carried on in the licensed premises only.

2. Each preparation manufactured shall be registered and shall bear a distinctive serial number, which shall be known as its batch number in the register in Form R.G.-3. This register shall also show the

receipt and disposal of all rectified spirit, opium, Indian hemp and other narcotic drugs and narcotics drawn from the spirit store and the quantity of finished preparation manufactured therefrom.

3. All finished preparations shall be transferred from the "laboratory" to the "finished store" and shall be so arranged that the checking of stock of every batch of preparation from the accounts register "in Form R.G.-4" is facilitated.

4. Finished preparations made from rectified spirit obtained at different rates of duty shall be kept separately in the finished store.

5. Every preparation stored in bulk shall be measured into the storage vessel to the nearest fluid ounce by the manufacturer and sealed.

6. When any of the contents of a vessel, in which the preparations are stored in bulk are removed, the manufacturer shall enter on the stock card attached thereto the quantity taken out and the manner of disposal with his signature and date.

Samples to be taken by the Excise Officer at least once a month for Analysis

1. The Excise Officer, in whose jurisdiction the manufactory is situated, shall, without previous notice to the manufacturer, take samples of not less than 13 percent, and not more than 15 per cent, (save in exceptional circumstances) of the total number of the medicinal and toilet preparations containing alcohol from the finished stocks at least once every month and forward them to the Chemical Examiner for analysis and report whether the alcoholic contents thereof tally with the percentage of alcohol shown on the labels affixed to the bottles.

2. If the proof strength reported by the Chemical Examiner is more than 3 percent. proof spirit than the strength declared by the manufacturer on the labels pasted on such bottles, the manufacturer is liable to a penalty at the rate of 10 times the difference in duty in the quantity so manufactured but not exceeding Rs. 2,000.

3. If such differences are found to occur frequently, the Excise Commissioner may order the cancellation of the licence held by the manufacturer.

4. Samples of finished products may also be taken at any time by the Excise Commissioner, and such other Excise Officer authorized by the Excise Commissioner in this behalf.

5. All such samples shall be taken by the officer personally and in the presence of the manufacturer or his authorized agent.

Procedure to be followed in taking samples

1. A sample shall be of 227 ml. or such quantity as may be fixed by the Excise Commissioner.

2. Every sample shall be taken in duplicate.

3. The cork of every bottle in which sample is kept shall be fixed with the officer's personal seal or the official seal and the name of the preparations and batch number shall be stated on label axed to each such bottle.

4. The label of the bottle shall be signed by the officer taking the sample.

5. The manufacturer, if he so desires shall be allowed to affix his own seal and sign the labels.

6. The duplicate samples shall be kept securely under lock and key in an almirah (to be provided by the manufacturer) until the result of the analysis has been reported, save in the case in which the Chemical Examiner has asked for another sample either to replace the previous sample dispatched to him or to repeat the analysis. Duplicate samples, to which no further reference is needed, shall be promptly returned to the manufacturer.

7. The samples to be sent for examination shall be carefully placed in a case and securely fastened with tape or wire to be supplied by the manufacturer and shall be sealed by the officer taking the samples, with the personal seal or the official seal, and dispatched without delay, at the expense of the manufacturer, to the Chemical Examiner.

8. A letter advising the dispatch of the sample shall be sent to the Chemical Examiner in duplicate. The letter shall contain besides other information a facsimile of the seal used. The Chemical Examiner

shall acknowledge the receipt of the sample in the duplicate copy to the dispatching officer.

No compensation to manufacturer of samples taken for analysis

The manufacturer shall not be entitled to any compensation for the samples taken for the purpose of analysis under these rules.

Correct and up-to-date accounts in prescribed printed registers to be maintained

1. The manufacturer shall maintain up-to-date, correct and proper accounts in the relevant register and deliver to the proper officer, by the 5th of each month, a monthly return of transactions of business.

2. The manufacturer shall also furnish such statements as may be required by the Excise Commissioner or by any officer empowered by him in this behalf.

3. All the account registers shall be obtained by the manufacturer at his cost from the respective Taluk office or Excise Office or such other office authorized to sell such registers.

Employees

1. The manufacturer shall furnish to the Excise Commissioner and the proper officer a list containing the names of the manager or assistant manager employed by him and of all other employees whose duties require them to another non-bonded manufactory.

2. He shall promptly inform the Excise Commissioner and the proper officer of any changes which he may choose to make in the list from time to time.

3. No person other than the person whose name is contained in the list shall enter the manufactory without the special permission of the proper officer.

Inspection

1. The non-bonded manufactory shall at all reasonable times by open to inspection by the Excise Commissioner and other Excise Officer having jurisdiction over the area in which the manufactory is situated.

2. The proper officer shall inspect the non-bonded manufactory at least once every month.

3. The State Government may authorize any officer of the prohibition, land revenue medical and public health department to inspect the non-bonded manufactory.

4.6 WAREHOUSING OF ALCOHOL PREPARATION

Ware housing of alcohol preparations are done in following manner-

1. **Establishment of bounded warehouses-** The manufacturers or dealers in dutiable goods may establish bonded warehouses anywhere in India. No duty paid goods and no goods other than dutiable goods shall be deposited in such bonded warehouses.

2. **Licensing of warehouses-** The Excise Commissioner shall licence a private warehouse for the storage of dutiable goods shall be stored and how and in what manner such warehouse shall be secured by locks or fastenings.

3. **Licensee to enter into a bond-** The Excise Commissioner shall require the licensee to furnish a bond in Form B-2 with such surety or sufficient security, in such amount and under such conditions, as the Excise Commissioner approves binding the licensee to pay duty on the goods deposited therein and for the due and sage removal of such goods to another warehouse and for the due observance of the terms, conditions and requirements of the Act, these rules and any other rule made hereunder in respect of the same.

Provided that on the revocation of any licence by the Excise Commissioner all such goods warehoused therein shall be removed as the Excise Commissioner directs and no abatement of duty or allowance shall be made in respect of any such goods for deficiency of quantity, strength or quality after due notice of such revocation has been given to the licensee;

Provided further that in the event of death, insolvency or insufficiency of the surety, the Excise Commissioner may, in his discretion, demand a fresh bond; and may, if the bond is with security, demand at any time he considers it fit to do so, additional security.

4. **Receipt of goods at warehouse-** All goods brought for warehousing shall be produced to the officer-in-charge of the warehouse, if any, or the proper officer, together with the relative transport and shall be weighed, gauged and proved, wherever necessary, in his presence and assessed to duty prior to entry into the warehouse and the quantity and description of the goods, the marks and numbers of the packages, the number and date of the permit and the amount of duty leviable thereon shall be noted in the warehouse register in Form R.G.-5. All goods received into the warehouse shall be kept separate from other goods until the receipt account has been taken by the officer-in charge or the proper officer as the case may be.

5. **Owner's power to deal with warehoused goods-** With the sanction of the officer-in-charge or the proper officer, as the case may be, and in accordance with such instructions as the Excise Commissioner may, from time to time, issue in writing in his behalf, any owner of goods lodged in a warehouse may sort, separate, pack and repack the goods and make such a alterations therein as may be necessary for the preservation, sale or disposal thereof. After the goods have been so separated and repacked in such manner, as may be ordered by the Excise Commissioner, the officer-incharge or the proper officer, as the case may be, may, at the owner's request, cause or permit any damaged goods remaining after such repacking to be destroyed subject to such limitations as the Excise Commissioner may, from time to time, impose and may remit the duty assessed thereon.

6. **Goods not to be taken out of warehouse except as provided by these Rules-** No goods shall be removed from any warehouse except on payment of duty or for removal to any other warehouse or for export and on presentation of a written application prescribed in rule 81 or rule 98, as the case may be.

7. **Periods for which goods may remain in warehouse under bond-** Any goods warehouse may be left in the warehouse in which they are deposited for a period of three years or such extended period as the Excise Commissioner in each case allow. The owner of any such goods remaining in the warehouse shall, before the expiry of

the period mentioned above, clear the same for consumption in the State after payment of duty or for removal in bond to another bonded warehouse or for exportation

8. **Mode for calculating quantity of goods warehouse-** The quantity of goods contained in any package warehouse may be calculated by weight, measure, gauge, proof strength, or in such other manner as the Excise Commissioner may direct.

9. **Power to remit duty on warehouse goods lost or destroyed-** If any goods lodged in a warehouse are lost or destroyed by unavoidable accident, the Excise Commissioner may remit the duty thereon.

   Provided that if any goods are so lost or destroyed, notice thereof shall be given to the officer-in-charge of the warehouse or the proper officer immediately on discovery of such loss or destruction.

10. **Responsibility of the licence of the warehouse-** The licensee of the warehouse in respect of goods lodged therein, shall be responsible for their due reception therein and delivery therefrom and for their safe custody while deposited therein, according to the quantity or weight reported by the officer who has assessed the goods.

11. **Offences with respect to warehousing-** If the owner by goods warehouse, by himself or by any person in his employ, or by any other person with his connivance commits any of the following offences, namely:

    a) Opens any of the locks or doors of the warehouse, which is required by these rules, or by any general or special order of the Excise

    b) Commissioner, to be locked or makes or obtains access into such a warehouse except in the presence of an office acting in his duty as such; or

    c) After the approval of a warehouse, makes any alternation therein or addition there to without the previous consent of the Excise Commissioner; or

    d) Warehouses goods in, or removes goods fro , a warehouse otherwise than as provided by these rules.

e)   privately removes or conceals any goods either before or after they are warehouse; he shall be liable to a penalty which may extend to two thousand rupees, and all goods warehouse, removed, or concealed in contravention of this rule shall be liable to confiscation.

12. **Monthly returns-**Which seven days after the close of each month, every licensee shall submit to the Excise Commissioner a monthly return showing the quantity of dutiable goods received, the quantity transferred to another warehouse under bond, the quantity removed on payment of duty and such other particulars as the State Government may be general or special order require.

13. **Clearance on payment of duty-** When the license desires to remove goods on payment of duty, he shall make an application in Form A.R.-2, in triplicate, to the officer-in-charge or the proper officer, as the case may be, at least twelve houses before he is intended to remove the goods. The officer shall, thereupon, assess the amount of duty leviable on the goods and on production of evidence that the sum has been paid into a treasury or the sum has been debited to the account-current, as the case may be, shall allow the goods to be cleared.

INTER-STATE TRANSPORT

Dutiable goods manufactured under bond or stored in a bonded warehouse in any State, unless exempted from payment of duty under rules 7 and 8, may be removed from such State to any other State,

1.   After payment of duty in the first mentioned State in the manner laid down in rule 40 or rule 81, as the case may be; or

2.   In bond, in the manner hereinafter prescribed for movement from one bonded warehouse to another.

4.7 TRANSPORT FROM ONE BONDED LABORATORY TO ANOTHER

Bond for due arrival and re-warehousing

1.   When warehoused goods are to be removed from one warehouse to another, the consignor or the consignee of the goods shall, before the goods are removed, enter into a bond in Form B-4 with such surety

or sufficient security as the Excise Commissioner may prescribe, for a sum equal, at least, to double the duty chargeable on such goods for the due arrival and rewarehousing thereof at the warehouse of destination within such time as the officer in charge of the warehouse of removal directs. Such bond shall be furnished to the officer in charge of the warehouse of removal, or of the warehouse of destination according as the bond is executed by the consignor or the consignee.

2. Such bond shall not be discharged until, such goods are produced to the officer at the warehouse of destination and are duly re-warehoused or are otherwise accounted for to the satisfaction of the State Excise Officer having jurisdiction over the executor of the bond nor until the full duty due upon any deficiency on such goods not so accounted for has been paid.

3. For purposes of such a discharge, if the bond has been furnished by the consignor, an essential condition shall be the prior receipt by the officer-in-charge of the warehouse of removal, of the duplicate application from the officer-in-charge of the warehouse of destination with his re-warehousing certificate recorded therein as hereinafter provided.

Remover may enter into a general bond

The Excise Commissioner may permit any person, to remove warehoused goods from one warehouse to another, by entering into a general bond in Form B-4, with such surety or sufficient security in such amount and under such condition, as the Excise Commissioner approves for the removal, from time to time, of any goods from one warehouse to another and for the due arrival and re-warehousing thereof at the warehouse of destination within such time as the officer-in-charge of the warehouse of removal directs :

Provided that in the event of death, insolvency of insufficiency of the surety, or when the amount of bond is inadequate the Excise Commissioner may, in his discretion, demand a fresh bond and may, if the bond is with security, demand at any time he considers fit to do so, additional security.

Procedure in respect of goods removed from one warehouse to another

1. The application for removal of goods from one warehouse to another in triplicate shall be presented by the consignor to the officer-in-charge of the warehouse removal at least 24 hours before the intended removal together with such other information as the Excise Commissioner may, by general or special rules or order, require.

2. Such officer shall then take account of the goods, and after completing the removal certificate on all the copies of the application, shall send the duplicate to the officer-in-charge of the warehouse of destination, and hand over the triplicate to the consignor for dispatch to the consignee. He shall also over-deliver to the consignor a transport permit.

3. On arrival of the goods at the warehouse of destination, the consignee shall present them together with the triplicate application and the transport permit to the officer-in-charge of such warehouse, who shall, after taking account of the goods, complete the re-warehousing certificate on the duplicate and the triplicate application and return the duplicate to the officer-in-charge of the warehouse of removal, and the triplicate to the consignee for dispatch to the consignor.

4. The consignor shall present the triplicate application duly endorsed with such certificate to the officer-in-charge of the warehouse of removal within ninety days of the date of issue of the transport permit.

Failure to present triplicate application

1. If the consignor fails to present the triplicate application to the officer-in-charge of the warehouse of removal in the manner laid down above, and the duplicate application endorsed with the rewarehousing certificate has also not been received by such officer, from the officer-in charge of the warehouse of destination, the consignor shall, upon a written demand being made by the former officer pay the duty leviable on such goods within ten days of the notice of demand and if the duty is not so paid, he shall not be permitted to make fresh removals of any warehoused goods from one warehouse to another until the duty is paid or until the triplicate application is so presented

or the duplicate application is so received.

2. Where such duty has been paid, it shall be refunded to the consignor, either on his presentation of his triplicate application to, or on the receipt of the duplicate application by the officer at the warehouse of removal, duly endorsed as provided above, with a certificate by the officer-in-charge of the warehouse of destination that the goods covered by the application have been satisfactorily re-warehoused.

Procedure on failure to pay duty

1. If the owner fails to pay any sum demanded under any of the preceding rules, the officer authorized in this behalf by the State Government may forthwith either proceed upon the bond executed by the owner of such goods, or cause such portion as he thinks fit of such goods (if any) in the warehouse, on account of which the money is due, to be detained with a view to recovering the demand; and if the demand is not discharged within ten days from the date of such detention, due notice thereof being given to the owner, the goods so detained may be sold by public auction duly advertised in the official Gazette, or in such other manner as the Excise Commissioner may, in any particular case direct.

2. The net proceeds of the sales of any goods so detained shall be adjusted against the amount due under the bond and the effect of such adjustment shall be recorded and if there is any surplus remaining after such adjustment, the surplus shall be paid to the owner of the goods :

Provided that application for the payment of such surplus is made within six months from the date of sale unless the period is extended by the Excise Commissioner on sufficient cause being shown.

4.8 EXPORT OF ALCOHOLIC PREPARATIONS

Method of export

Duty-paid goods shall be exported under claim for rebate of duty. Goods under bond for payment of duty shall be sent to the place of export under bond for their due export.

Application to be submitted

The exporter shall present to the officer incharge or the proper officer, as the case may be, an application in triplicate in Form A.R.-3 if the goods are to be exported by land and in Form A.R.-4 if the goods are to be exported by sea or air or by parcel post. The officer-in-charge or the proper officer shall send the original to the customs officer or the border examiner or the postmaster, as the case may be, at the place of export, deliver the duplicate to the consignor and retain the triplicate as office copy. A separate application shall be submitted in respect of each consignment.

Examination of goods prior to despatch

1. **Goods under bond-** When goods from a bonded manufactory or warehouse are to be exported, the cases or packages, in which such goods are packed, shall be legibly marked in ink or oil colour (or in such other durable manner as the Excise Commissioner may in any particular case allow), with a progressive number commencing with No. 1 for each year, with the owner's name and special mark, if any, the total quantity of dutiable goods with their alcoholic contents in London-proof litres.

2. **Duty paid goods-** The owner of a non-bonded manufactory or a wholesale dealer, who wants to export duty paid goods shall give 48 hours' notice to the proper officer, for supervising packing of the goods to be exported. The manufacturer or wholesale dealer shall present the entire consignment to be exported to the proper officer. The said officer shall take samples from each kind of dutiable goods to be exported and shall allow the dispatch of the goods subject to fulfilling further conditions laid down in sub-rule (3). Thereafter shall send the samples to the Chemical Examiner for analysis. On receipt of the analysis report of the Chemical Examiner, the proper officer shall enter the alcoholic content in London-proof litres of the goods packed as ascertained by analysis in the duplicate copy of the application which the owner shall present to him before its presentation to the Excise Commissioner for claiming rebate of excise duty as laid down in rule 103,

Provided that the process of determining alcoholic content by chemical analysis shall be dispensed with in the case of goods sent out from a bonded manufactory or warehouse it the owner of such goods chooses to pay the duty on goods to be exported in lieu of entering into a bond for due transport of goods to the place of report and in which case the procedure laid down in sub-rule (1) shall apply.

3. After verifying the particulars entered in the application, and, in the case duty-paid goods, after satisfying himself that the goods are identifiable as the goods, in respect of which the payment of duty cited in the application was made, the officer-incharge or the proper officer, as the case may be, shall get the following particulars noted in the body of each package :

a. Name and address of the consignee.

b. Description of the goods,

c. Total quantity of the goods packed.

d. Alcoholic content of the goods in London-proof litres as declared by the manufacturer,

e. Gross weight of the package, and shall then sell each package with his official seal in such a manner that the package cannot be tampered with without breaking the seal. The said officer shall endorse all copies of the application, shall specify the period within which the goods shall be actually exported and return the duplicate to the consignor, who, after dispatching the goods shall enter the number and date of the railway receipt or bill of lading in the duplicate copy and shall communicate these particulars to the proper officer for entry in the other copies.

Examination at the place of export

On arrival at the place of export by post have been sealed, the exporter shall present the duplicate application, together with the packet or packets to which it refers, to the postmaster at the office of booking.

Examination at the place of export

On arrival at the place of export, the goods shall be presented, together with the duplicate application, to the Customs Collection Border Examiner, or any officer, of customs or land customs duly appointed for the purpose. The consignment shall be carefully examined and check-weighed and if the seals are intact and the case or the packages correspond with the description given in the application, and the particulars stated in the duplicate application and the original received from the officer at the place of dispatch agree in all respects, the Customs Collector, Border Examiner, or any such officer of customs shall allow export and shall then certify on the duplicate application that the goods have been duly exported (citing in the case of exports by sea or air, the shipping bill number and date and other particulars of export) and return it to the exporter.

Further procedure in respect of goods exported by parcel post

Where the goods are exported by post, the postmaster of the post office of final dispatch from India shall certify on the duplicate application that the goods covered by the application have been duly exported out of India and shall return it, through the postmaster at the post office of booking, to the exporter. The original application shall be returned to the officer-in-charge of the proper officer with the certificate of export.

Presentation of claim for rebate

In order to obtain payment of the rebate, the exporter shall produce to the Excise Commissioner from whose jurisdiction the goods were dispatched, the duplicate application bearing the certificate of the officer, who examined the goods at the port or post office of export or the frontier, as the case may be. If the Excise Commissioner is satisfied from comparison of the duplicate application with the original received from such certifying officer, that the claim is in order, he shall sanction the rebate,

Provided such claims for rebate of duty shall be made within one month from the date of issue of the certificate of the officer who examined the goods at the port or post office of export or the frontier, as the case may be,

Provided further that the Excise Commissioner may in his discretion extend the period within such claims for rebate shall be made.

4.9   POWERS, DUTIES AND RESPONSIBILITIES OF EXCISE OFFICER

Power to arrest

1.   Any excise officer duly empowered by rules made in this behalf may arrest any person whom he has reason to believe to be liable to punishment under this Act.

2.   Any person accused or reasonably suspected of committing an offence under this Act or any rules made thereunder, who, on demand of any excise officer duly empowered by rules made under this Act, refuses to give his name and residence, or who gives a name or residence which such officer has reason to believe to be false may be arrested by such officer in order that his name and residence may be ascertained.

Power to summon persons to give evidence and produce documents in inquiries under this Act

1.   Any excise officer duly empowered by rules made in this behalf shall have power to summon any person whose attendance he considers necessary either to give evidence or to produce a document or any other thing in any inquiry whichsuch officer is making for any of the purpose of this Act.

2.   A summons to produce documents or other things under sub-section (1) may be for the production of certain specified documents or things or for the production of all documents or things of a certain description in the possession or under the control of the person concerned.

3.   All persons so summoned shall be bound to attend either in person or by an authorized agent as such officer may direct and all persons so summoned shall be bound to state the truth on any subject

respecting which he is examined or make statements and produce such documents and other things as may be required:

Provided that the exemption under Sec. 132 and Sec. 133 of the Code of Civil Procedure, 1908 (5 of 1908), shall apply to requisitions for attendance under this section.

4.   Every such inquiry as aforesaid shall be deemed to be a judicial proceeding within the meaning of Sec. 193 and Sec. 228 of the Indian Penal Code (45 of 1860).

Officers are required to assist Excise officers

All officers of Customs and Central Excise, and such other officers of the Central Government as may be specified in this behalf, and all police officers and all officers engaged in the collection of land revenue are hereby empowered and required to assist excise officers in the execution of this Act.

Punishment for connivance at offences

Any owner or occupier of land or any agent of such owner or occupier in charge of the management of the land, who wilfully connives at any offence against the provisions of this Act or any rules made thereunder shall, for every such offence, be punishable with imprisonment for a term which may extend to six months, or with fine which may extend to five hundred rupees, or with both.

Searches and arrests how to be made

All arrests and searches made under this Act or under any rules made thereunder shall be carried out in accordance with the provisions of the Code of Criminal Procedure, 1895 (5 of 1898), relating respectively to searches and arrests under the Code.

Disposal of persons arrested

1.   Every person arrested under this Act shall be forwarded without delay to the nearest Excise Officer empowered to send persons so arrested to a Magistrate or if there is no such excise officer within a reasonable distance to the officer-in-charge of the nearest police station.

2. The officer-in-charge of a police station to whom any person is forwarded under sub-section (1) shall either admit him to bail to appear before a Magistrate having jurisdiction or in default of bail forward him without delay in custody to such Magistrate.

Inquiry how to be made by excise officers against arrested persons forwarded to them

1. When any person is forwarded under Sec. 15 to an excise officer empowered to send persons so arrested to a Magistrate, the Excise Officer shall proceed to inquire into the charge against him.

2. For the purpose of sub-section (1), the Excise Officer may exercise the same powers, and shall be subject to the same provisions, as the officer-in-charge of a police station may exercise and is subject to under the Code of Criminal Procedure, 1895 (5 of 1898), when investigating a cognizable case.

Provided that –

a. If the Excise Officer is of opinion that there is sufficient evidence or reasonable ground of suspicion against the accused person he shall either admit him to bail to appear before Magistrate having jurisdiction in the case, or forward him in custody without delay to such Magistrate;

b. If it appears to the Excise Officer that there is not sufficient evidence or reasonable ground of suspicion against the accused person, he shall release the accused person on his executing a bond with or without sureties as the Excise Officer may direct, to appear, if and when so required, before the Magistrate having jurisdiction and shall make a full report of all the particulars of the case to his official superior.

c. All officers exercising any powers under Sec. 15 or this section shall so exercise their powers as to ensure that every person who is arrested and detained in custody is produced before the nearest Magistrate within a period of twenty-four hours of such arrest excluding the time necessary for the journey from the place of arrest to the Court of the Magistrate.

Vexatious search, seizure, etc. by Excise Officer

1. Any officer exercising powers under this Act or under the rules made thereunder who-

    a. Without reasonable ground of suspicion searches or causes to be searched any place, conveyance or vessel;

    b. Vexatiously and unnecessarily detains searches or arrests any person;

    c. Vexatiously and unnecessarily seizes the moveable property of any person on pretence of seizing or searching for any article liable to confiscation under this Act;

    d. Commits, as such officer, any other act to the injury of any person, without having reason to believe that such act is required for the execution of his duty; shall, for every such offence, be punishable with fine which may extend to two thousand rupees.

2. Any person wilfully and maliciously giving false information and so causing an arrest or a search to be made under this Act shall be punishable with imprisonment for a term which may extend to two years, or with fine which may extend to two thousand rupees, or with both.

Failure of excise officers on duty

An Excise Officer who ceases or refuses to perform, or withdraws himself from the duties of his office, unless he had obtained the express written permission of his superior officer or has given such superior officer two months' notice in writing of his intention or has other lawful excuse, shall be punishable with imprisonment for a term which may extend to three months, or with fine which may extend to three months' pay, or with both.

Authorized officers to have free access to premises, equipment, stocks and accounts of dealers in dutiable goods

Any officer authorized in writing by the Excise Commissioner in this behalf, shall have free access at all reasonable timers to any premises licensed under these rules and to any place where dutiable goods are manufactured, stored or kept for sale, and may, with or without notice to the owner, inspect the building, the plant, the machinery, the stocks and the accounts, and may at any time check the records made of the goods stocked in, or removed from the manufactory, warehouse or place of their transfer within a manufactory to that part of the premises, if any, in which they are to be used for the manufacture of any other commodity, whether for the purpose of testing the accuracy of any return submitted under these rules, or of informing himself as to any particulars regarding which information is required for the purpose of the Act or these rules.

Penalty for obstruction or for giving false or misleading information

If any person by himself or by any person in his employ-

1. Voluntarily obstructs or offers any resistance to or impedes, or otherwise interferes with; or

2. Wilfully gives false or misleading information to the officer duly appointed under rule 110, who is acting in accordance with his duty thereunder; such person shall be liable to a penalty which may extend to five hundred rupees.

Power to detain person and examine goods

Any Excise Officer duly empowered by the State Government may stop and detain any person found carrying or removing any dutiable goods for the transport of which a permit or other transport document is required by these rules, and may examine the goods and may require the production of a permit or other document authorizing the removal thereof. If a permit or other prescribed document is produced agreeing with the goods in all respects, the officer may endorse thereon the time and place of his examination thereof.

Power to stop, enter and search

Any Excise Officer not below the rank of a sub-inspector of excise may stop and search any vessel, car or other means of conveyance for dutiable goods, and enter and search at any time by day or by night and land, building any enclosed place, premises, vessel, conveyance or other place upon or in which he has reason to believe that dutiable goods are stored, manufactured or carried or in contravention of the provisions of the Act or these rules, and in case of resistance break open any door and remove any other obstacle to his entry, and search into such land, building and closed places, premises, vessel, conveyance or other place.

Seizure

Any Excise Officer not below the rank of a sub-inspector of excise may seize and remove or detain any goods in respect of which, it appears to him, the duty should have been, but has not been, levied or that contravention of the provisions of the Act or these rules has occurred. He may also seize and remove or detain any receptacle, packages or coverings, in which such goods or articles are contained, and animals, vehicles, vessels or other conveyances used in carrying such goods or articles and any implements and machinery used in the manufacture of such goods.

Power to require access to place, vessel or conveyance for inspection or examination of goods

Any officer not below the rank of a sub-inspector of excise may require any person who has the immediate possession, control or use of any land, building, enclosed place, premises, vessel, conveyance or other place which he desires to search under these rules, or of any dutiable goods, stored manufactured or carried thereupon or therein, to open or allow access to inspect or examine such place or conveyance or to open, unload, unpack or allow the inspection or examination of such articles.

Police to take charge of articles seized

All officers-in charge of police stations shall take charge of and keep in safe custody, pending the orders of the Magistrate or of the adjudicating Excise Officer, all things seized under the Act or these rules which may be delivered to them, and shall allow any officer who may accompany such goods to the police or who may be deputed for the purpose by his superior officer, to affix his seal to such things or to take samples of and from them. All samples so taken shall also be sealed with the seal of the officer-in-charge of the police station.

Summons and notices (Manner of service)

1. Any Excise Officer not below the rank of a sub-inspector of excise may summon any person whose attendance he considers necessary either to give evidence or to produce documents or any other things, in any enquiry which such officer is making for any of the purposes of the Act or the rules.

2. Every summon or notice issued under the Act or the rules shall be in writing in duplicate, and shall state the purpose for which it is issued, and shall be signed by the officer issuing it, and shall also bear his official seal, if he has any; and shall be served by tendering a copy of it to the person summoned, or if he cannot be found, by affixing a copy of it to some conspicuous part of the house in which he is known to have last resided, or carried on business or personally worked for gain.

Service of notice (Notice not void for error)

No notice shall be deemed void on account of an error in the name or designation of any person referred to therein, unless such error has produced a material misconception of the intended intimation.

Disposal of things seized

1. The owner or person having the charge of any animal seized and detained shall provide from day to day for its keep while detained, and if he fails to do so, such animal may be sold by public auction, and the expenses (if any) incurred on account of it defrayed from the proceeds of the sale.

2. When anything is seized an order for its release is subsequently passed and owner does not, within a period of one month, appear to claim such thing and tender the duties, penalties and charge (if any) due in respect thereof, it may be sold by public auction; and such duties, penalties, and charges will be defrayed from the proceeds of the sale.

3. Surplus proceeds of a sale under these rules shall, if not claimed by the owner of the things seized within a period of three months from the date of such sale be forfeited, to the collecting Government.

Prosecution

No prosecutions under the Act shall be instituted except by an Excise Officer not below the rank of a sub-inspector of excise.

Arrests

Any Excise Officer not below the rank of a sub-inspector of excise may arrest any person whom he has reason to believe to be liable to punishment under the Act or any person who, on demand by him refuse to give his name and residence, or who gives his name and address which such officer has reason to believe to be false.

Provisions of arrests and seizures to be in conformity with the Act

All arrests and seizures made under these rules shall be in conformity with the provisions of the Act and the rules.

4.10 OFFENCES AND PENALTIES

S.no	OFFENCES	PENALTIES
1	Failure to follow the condition of licence or pay duty or manufacture dutiable goods without licence or provide false information.	Six months imprisonment or Rs 2000/- fine or both.
2	Any owner or occupier of the land who wilfully connives at the commission of an offence.	Six months imprisonment or Rs 500/- fine or both.
3	Any person who wilfully and maliciously gives false information.	Two years imprisonment or Rs 2000/- fine or both.

Continued on Next Page

S.no	OFFENCES	PENALTIES
4	Any person who makes false entries or tears out pages from the stock book.	Fine up to Rs 2000/-.
5	Dutiable goods not stored in an orderly manner as directed.	Fine up to Rs 1000/-.
6	Dutiable goods are not wrapped or labelled as prescribed.	Fine up to Rs 1000/-.
7	A person authorised to export dutiable goods under bond fails to furnish proof of export.	Duty plus fine up to Rs 2000/-.
8	a)Open lock or door of warehouse. b)Make any alteration in the warehouse. c) Remove ant goods in contravention of the rules.	Fine up to Rs 2000/-.
9	Anyone who obstructs or resists or give any false or misleading information.	Fine up to Rs 5000/-.
10	An officer of the excise department who unnecessarily detains searches or arrests or seizes any property.	Fine up to Rs 2000/-.
11	Any excise officer who ceases or refuses to do his duty.	Three months imprisonment or fine up to three months or both.
12	If any excise officer discloses information acquired in the course of his duty.	Fine up to Rs 1000/-.

REVIEW QUESTIONS

ESSAY QUESTIONS

1. Write a note on licensing procedure under Medicinal and Toilet preparation Act 1955.

2. Explain in detail requirements and procedure for manufacturing of Medicinal and Toilet preparations in bond.

3. Explain in detail requirements and procedure for manufacturing of Medicinal and Toilet preparations manufacturing outside bond.

SHORT QUESTIONS

1. Define.

   a) Alcohol.

   b) Dutiable goods.

   c) Medicinal preparations.

   d) Toilet preparations.

   e) Bonded laboratories.

   f) Non-bonded laboratories.

   g) Denatured alcohol.

   h) Absolute alcohol.

2. What are the objectives of Medicinal and Toilet preparation act 1955?

3. Write a note on warehousing of Alcoholic preparations.

4. Write a note on export of Alcoholic preparations.

5. Write a note on Interstate transport of Alcoholic goods.

6. Explain the Powers, Duties and Responsibilities of Excise Officer.

7.   What are the various offences and penalties under the Medicinal
       and Toilet preparation Act 1955?

MCQ's

1.   Which of the following is not associated with Medicinal and Toilet
       preparation Act?

       a.   1955.

       b.   1967.

       c.   1975.

       d.   1976.

2.   Manufacture outside the bond is also called as,

       a.   Manufacture in bond.

       b.   Manufacture without the bond.

       c.   Bonded laboratories.

       d.   Non-bonded laboratories.

3.   Which one of the following is not a power of excise officer?

       a.   Inspection.

       b.   Search.

       c.   Suspension of licence.

       d.   Countersigning the indent.

4.   "The excise officer in a case of offence forwards the articles
       seized to the officer in charge of police station". What is the excise
       officer performing in this act?

       a.   Duty.

       b.   Power.

       c.   Responsibility.

d.   None of the above.

5.   Inspection is must in,

a.   Bonded laboratories.

b.   Non-bonded laboratories.

c.   Both (a) and (b).

d.   None of the above.

6.   In which of the following case alcoholic preparation can be exported from India?

a.   Export under bond.

b.   Export after payment of duty.

c.   None of the above.

d.   Both (a) and (b).

Answers: 1-b, 2-b &d, 3-d, 4-c, 5-b, 6-d.

Chapter 5

NARCOTIC DRUGS AND PSYCHOTROPIC SUBSTANCES ACT 1985

5.1 INTRODUCTION

It is an Act to consolidate and amend the law relating to narcotic drugs, to make stringent provisions for the control and regulation of operations relating to narcotic drugs and psychotropic substances to provide for the forfeiture of property derived from, or used in, illicit traffic in narcotic drugs and psychotropic substances, to implement the provisions of the International Conventions on Narcotic Drugs and Psychotropic Substances and for matters connected therewith.

Natural drugs like coca, opium and hemp though excellent drugs have a drawback of habit forming. These drugs are used to satisfy addiction and luxury. These drugs cause hallucination and excessive use of them causes physical and mental injury, producing moral weakness and lack of sense of self-respect.

Due to all these degenerative effects of these drugs, Governments of different countries have restricted their use strictly for medical use only.

The cultivation of Opium (poppy) was brought under control in India in 1857, and this was supplemented by Opium Act 1878. With the confirmation of Geneva Convention the Dangerous Drug Act, 1930 was passed by the Indian Legislature.

In spite of these laws, there is continued use of natural and synthetic drugs for the purpose of addiction. With reference to Opium Act and Dangerous Drugs Act, the penalties charged in India were very low as compared to other countries. So to make stringent and uniform provisions exemplary (increased) punishment was provided for most of the offences. To curb the same effectively the Narcotic Drugs and Psychotropic Substance act 1985 was passed. This act repealed the two Opium Acts (1857, 1878) and the Dangerous Drug Act 1930.

5.2 DEFINITIONS

1. *Addict:* Means a person addicted to any narcotic drug or psychotropic substance.

2. *Cannabis (hemp):* Means –

    a)   Charas- the separated resin, in whatever form, whether crude or purified, obtained from the cannabis plant and also includes concentrated preparation and resin known as hashish oil or liquid hashish.

    b)   Ganja- the flowering or fruiting tops of the cannabis plant (excluding the seeds and leaves when not accompanied by the tops), by whatever name they may be known or designated; and

    c)   Any mixture, with or without any neutral material, of any of the above forms of cannabis or any drink prepared there from.

3. *Cannabis plant:* Means any plant of the genus cannabis.

4. *Coca derivative:* Means –

    a)   Crude cocaine, that is, any extract of coca leaf which can be used, directly or indirectly, for the manufacture of cocaine.

    b)   Ecgonine and all the derivatives of ecgonine from which it can be recovered.

    c)   Cocaine, that is, methyl ester of benzoyl-ecgonine and its salts; and

    d)   All preparations containing more than 0.1 % of cocaine.

5. *Coca leaf:* Means –

    a)   The leaf of the coca plant except a leaf from which all ecgonine, cocaine and any other ecgonine alkaloids have been removed.

b) Any mixture thereof with or without any neutral material, out does not include any preparation containing not more than 0.1 % of cocaine.

6. *Coca plant:* Means the plant of any species of the genus Frythroxylon.

7. *Controlled substance:* Means any substance which the Central Government may, having regard to the available information as to its possible use in the production or manufacture of narcotic drugs or psychotropic substances or to the provisions of any International Convention, by notification in the Official Gazette, declare to be a controlled substance,

8. *Illicit traffic:* In relation to narcotic drugs and psychotropic substances, means –

a) Cultivating any coca plant or gathering any portion of coca plant.

b) Cultivating the opium poppy or any cannabis plant.

c) Engaging in the production, manufacture, possession, sale, purchase, transportation, warehousing, concealment, use or consumption, import inter-State, export inter-State, import into India, and export from India or transhipment, of narcotic drugs or psychotropic substances.

d) Dealing in any activities in narcotic drugs or psychotropic substances other than those referred to in sub-clauses (i) to (ii); or

e) Handling or letting out any premises for the carrying on of any of the activities referred to in sub-clauses (i) to (iv), other than those permitted under this Act, or any rule or order made, or any condition of any licence, term or authorisation issued, there under, and includes –

➢ Financing, directly or indirectly, any of the aforementioned activities.

➢ Abetting or conspiring in the furtherance of or in support of doing any of the aforementioned activities; and

➢ Harbouring persons engaged in any of the aforementioned activities.

9. *Manufacture:* In relation to narcotic drugs or psychotropic substances, includes –

a) All processes other than production by which such drugs or substances may be obtained.

b) Refining of such drugs or substances.

c) Transformation of such drugs or substances; and

d) Making of preparation with or containing such drugs or substances.

10. *Manufactured drug:* Means –

a) All coca derivatives, medicinal cannabis, opium derivatives and poppy straw concentrate.

b) Any other narcotic substance or preparation which the Central Government may, having regard to the available information as to its nature or to a decision, if any, under any International Convention, by notification in the Official Gazette, declare not to be a manufactured drug.

11. *Medicinal cannabis:* Means medicinal hemp means any extract or tincture of cannabis (hemp).

12. *Narcotics Commissioner:* Means the Narcotics Commissioner appointed under section 5.

13. *Narcotic drug:* Means coca leaf, cannabis (hemp), opium, poppy straw and includes all manufactured drugs.

14. *Opium:* Means –

a) The coagulated juice of the opium poppy; and

b) Any mixture, with or without any neutral material, of the coagulated juice of the opium poppy, but does not include any preparation containing not more than 0.2 % of morphine.

15. Opium Derivative: Means –

a) Medicinal opium, that is, opium which has undergone the processes necessary to adapt it for medicinal use in accordance with the requirements of the Indian Pharmacopoeia or any other pharmacopoeia notified in this behalf by the Central Government, whether in powder form or granulated or otherwise or mixed with neutral materials.

b) Prepared opium, that is, any product of opium obtained by any series of operations designed to transform opium into an extract suitable for smoking and the dross or other residue remaining after opium is smoked.

c) Phenanthrene alkaloids, namely, morphine, codeine, thebaine and their salts.

d) diacetylmorphine, that is, the alkaloid also known as diamorphine or heroin and its salts; and

e) All preparations containing more than 0.2 % of morphine or containing any diacetylmorphine.

16. Opium poppy: Means –

a) The plant of the species Papaver somniferum L; and

b) The plant of any other species of Papaver from which opium or any phenanthrene alkaloid can be extracted and which the Central Government may, by notification in the Official Gazette, declare to be opium poppy for the purposes of this Act.

17. Poppy straw: Means all parts (except the seeds) of the opium poppy after harvesting whether in their original form or cut, crushed or powdered and whether or not juice has been extracted therefrom.

18. ***Poppy straw concentrate:*** Means the material arising when poppy straw has entered into a process for the concentration of its alkaloids.

19. ***Psychotropic substance:*** Means any substance, natural or synthetic, or any natural material or any salt or preparation of such substance or material included in the list of psychotropic substances specified in the Schedule.

5.3 ADMINISTRATION OF THE ACT

1. ADVISORY (Consultative Committee)

1. The Central Government may constitute, by notification in the Official Gazette, an advisory committee to be called "The Narcotic Drugs and Psychotropic Substances Consultative Committee" to advise the Central Government on such matters relating to the administration of this Act as are referred to it by that Government from time to time.

2. The Committee shall consist of a Chairman and such other members, not exceeding twenty, as may be appointed by the Central Government.

3. The Committee shall meet when required to do so by the Central Government and shall have power to regulate its own procedure.

4. The Committee may, if it deems it necessary so to do for the efficient discharge of any of its functions, constitute one or more sub-committees and may appoint to any such sub-committee, whether generally or for the consideration of any particular matter, any person (including a non-official) who is not a member of the Committee.

5. The term of office of, the manner of filling casual vacancies in the offices of and the allowances, if any, payable to, the Chairman and other members of the Committee, and the conditions and restrictions subject to which the Committee may appoint a person who is not a member of the Committee as a member of any of its sub-committees, shall be such as may be prescribed by rules made by the Central Government.

2. EXECTUTIVE (Narcotic Commissioner)

Officers of Central Government

1. The Central Government shall appoint a Narcotics Commissioner and may also appoint such other officers with such designations as it thinks fit for the purposes of this Act.

2. The Narcotics Commissioner shall, either by himself or through officers subordinate to him, exercise all powers and perform all functions relating to the superintendence of the cultivation of the opium poppy and production of opium and shall also exercise and perform such other powers and functions as may be entrusted to him by the Central Government.

3. The officers appointed under sub-section (1) shall be subject to the general control and direction of the Central Government, or, if so directed by that Government, also of the Board or any other authority or officer.

Officers of State Government

1. The State Government may appoint such officers with such designations as it thinks fit for the purposes of this Act.

2. The officers appointed under sub-section (1) shall be subject to the general control and direction of the State Government, or, if so directed by that Government, also of any other authority or officer.

5.4 PROHIBITIONS

No person shall –

1. Cultivate any coca plant or gather any portion of coca plant; or

2. Cultivate the opium poppy or any cannabis plant; or

3. Produce, manufacture, possess, sell, purchase, transport, warehouse, use, consume, import inter-State, export inter-State, import into India, export from India or tranship any narcotic drug or psychotropic substance, except for medical or scientific

purposes and in the manner and to the extent provided by the provisions of this Act or the rules or orders made there under and in a case where any such provision, imposes any requirement by way of licence, permit or authorisation also in accordance with the terms and conditions of such licence, permit or authorisation; or

4. Convert or transfer any property if it is derived for an offence committed under this act or other corresponding law of any other country or from an act of participation in such offence or to assist any person in the commission of an offence; or

5. Conceal or disguise the true nature, source, location, disposition of any property knowing that such property is derived from an offence corresponding law of any other country; or

6. Knowingly acquire, possess or use any property which was derived from an offence committed under this act or under any other corresponding law of any other country.

Provided that, and subject to the other provisions of this Act and the rules made thereunder, the prohibition against the cultivation of the cannabis plant for the production of ganja or the production, possession, use, consumption, purchase, sale, transport, warehousing, import inter-State and export inter-State of ganja for any purpose other than medical and scientific purpose shall take effect only from the date which the Central Government may, by notification in the Official Gazette, specify in this behalf.

Provided further that, nothing in this section shall apply to the export of poppy straw for decorative purposes.

5.5 POWER OF CENTRAL GOVERNMENT TO PERMIT, CONTROL AND REGULATE

1. The Central Government may, by rules permit and regulate –

a) The cultivation, or gathering of any portion (such cultivation or gathering being only on account of the Central Government) of coca plant, or the production, possession, sale, purchase, transport, import inter-State, export inter-State, use or consumption of coca leaves.

b) The cultivation (such cultivation being only on account of Central Government) of the opium poppy.

c) The production and manufacture of opium and production of poppy straw.

d) The sale of opium and opium derivatives from the Central Government factories for export from India or sale to State Government or to

e) Manufacturing chemists.

f) The manufacture of manufactured drugs (other than prepared opium) but not including manufacture of medicinal opium or any preparation containing any manufactured drug from materials which the maker is lawfully entitled to possess.

g) The manufacture, possession, transport, imports inter-State, export inter-State, sale, purchase, consumption or use of psychotropic substances.

h) The import into India and export from India and transhipment of narcotic drugs and psychotropic substances;

i) Prescribe any other matter requisite to render effective the control of the Central Government over any of the matters specified in clause (a).

2. In particular and without prejudice to the generality of the foregoing power, such rules may –

a) Empower the Central Government to fix from time to time the limits within which licenses may be given for the cultivation of the opium poppy.

b) Require that all opium, the producer of land cultivated with the opium poppy, shall be delivered by the cultivators to the officers authorised in this behalf by the Central Government.

c) Prescribe the forms and conditions of licences for cultivation of the opium poppy and for production and manufacture of opium; the fees that may be charged therefore; the authorities by which such licences may be granted, withheld, refused or cancelled and the authorities before which appeals against the orders of withholding, refusal or cancellation of licences shall lie.

d) Prescribe that opium shall be weighed, examined and classified according to its quality and consistence by the officers authorised in this behalf by the Central Government in the presence of the cultivator at the time of delivery by the cultivator.

e) Empower the Central Government to fix from time to time the price to be paid to the cultivators for the opium delivered.

f) Provide for the weighment, examination and classification, according to the quality and consistence, of the opium received at the factory and the deductions from or additions (if any) to the standard price to be made in accordance with the result of such examination; and the authorities by which the decisions with regard to the weighment, examination, classification, deductions or additions shall be made and the authorities before which appeals against such decisions shall lie.

g) Require that opium delivered by a cultivator, if found as a result of examination in the Central Government factory to be adulterated, may be confiscated by the officers authorised in this behalf.

h) Prescribe the forms and conditions of licences for the manufacture of manufactured drugs, the authorities by which such licences may be granted and the fees that may be charged therefore.

i) Prescribe the forms and conditions of licences or permits for the manufacture, possession, transport, import inter-State, export inter-State, sale, purchase, consumption or use of psychotropic substances, the authorities by which such licences or permits may be granted and the fees that may be charged therefore.

j) Prescribe the ports and other places at which any kind of narcotic drugs or psychotropic substances may be imported into India or exported from India or transhipped; the forms and conditions of certificates, authorisations or permits, as the case may be, for such import, export or transhipment; the authorities by which such certificates, authorisations or permits may be granted and the fees that may be charged therefore.

POWER TO CONTROL AND REGULATE CONTROLLED SUBSTANCES

1. If the Central Government is of the opinion that, having regard to the use of any controlled substance in the production or manufacture of any narcotic drug or psychotropic substance, it is necessary or expedient so to do in the public interest, it may, by order, provide for regulating or prohibiting the production, manufacture, supply and distribution thereof and trade and commerce therein.

2. Without prejudice to the generality of the power conferred by sub-section (1), an order made there under may provide for regulating by licences, permits or otherwise, the production, manufacture, possession, transport, import inter-State, export inter-State, sale, purchase, consumption, use, storage, distribution, disposal or acquisition of any controlled substance.

5.6 POWER OF STATE GOVERNMENT TO PERMIT, CONTROL AND REGULATE

1. Subject to the provisions of section 8, the State Government may, by rules permit and regulate –

a) The possession, transport, imports inter-State, export inter-State, warehousing, sale, purchase, consumption and use of poppy straw.

b) The possession, transport, imports inter-State, export inter-State, sale, purchase, consumption and use of opium.

c) The cultivation of any cannabis plant, production, manufacture, possession, transport, import inter-State, export inter-State, sale, purchase, consumption or use of cannabis (excluding charas).

d) The manufacture of medicinal opium or any preparation containing any manufactured drug from materials which the maker is lawfully entitled to possess.

e) The possession, transport, purchase, sale, import inter-State, export inter-State, use or consumption of manufactured drugs other than prepared opium and of coca leaf and any preparation containing any manufactured drug.

f) The manufacture and possession of prepared opium from opium lawfully possessed by an addict registered with the State Government on medical advice for his personal consumption.

Provided that save in so far as may be expressly provided in the rules made under sub-clauses (iv) and (v), nothing in section 8 shall apply to the import inter-State, export inter-State, transport, possession, purchase, sale, use or consumption of manufactured drugs which are the property and in the possession of the Government:

Provided further that such drugs as are referred to in the preceding proviso shall not be sold or otherwise delivered to any person who, under the rules made by the State Government under the aforesaid sub-clauses, is not entitled to their possession;

g) Prescribe any other matter requisite to render effective the control of the State Government over any of the matters specified in clause (a).

2. In particular and without prejudice to the generality of the foregoing power, such rules may-

a) Empower the State Government to declare any place to be warehouse wherein it shall be the duty of the owners to deposit all such poppy straw as is legally imported inter-State and is intended for export inter-State or export from India; to regulate the safe custody of such poppy straw warehoused and the removal of such poppy straw for sale or export inter-State or export from India; to levy fees for such warehousing and to prescribe the manner in which and the period after which the poppy straw warehoused shall be disposed of in default of payment of fees.

b) Provide that the limits within which licences may be given for the cultivation of any cannabis plant shall be fixed from time to time by or under the orders of the State Government.

c) Provide that only the cultivators licensed by the prescribed authority of the State Government shall be authorized to engage in cultivation of any cannabis plant.

d) Require that all cannabis, the producer of land cultivated with cannabis plant, shall be delivered by the cultivators to the officers of the State Government authorized in this behalf.

e) Empower the State Government to fix from time to time, the price to be paid to the cultivators for the cannabis delivered.

f) Prescribe the forms and conditions of licences or permits for the purposes specified in sub-clauses (i) to (vi) of clause (a) of subsection (1) and the authorities by which such licences or permits may be granted and the fees that may be charged therefor.

5.7 SPECIAL PROVISIONS

A. REGARDING CULTIVATION OF OPIUM

1. The opium can be cultivated only on behalf of the central government, under a licence.

2. The licence of cultivation of opium poppy granted by the district opium officer on payment of Rs 25/- fees.

3. The licence specifies the area and designates the plots to be cultivated.

4. District Opium Officer appoints a cultivator as Lambardar in each village, who performs functions specified by Narcotic Commissioner.

5. The licence may be withheld or cancelled by higher rank officer.

6.   If licence is withheld or cancelled, the standing crop may be destroyed.

B. REGARDING PRODUCTION OF OPIUM

1.   During the course of harvesting, the cultivator should take each day's collection to Lambardar for weighment and make entry in record and attested jointly.

2.   All opium produced is delivered to District Opium Officer, who will weigh, examine and classify.

3.   All collected Opium is sent to the Government Opium Factor and classified by its general manager.

4.   If Opium is found to be adulterated, it is liable to confiscation.

5.   The Central Government from time to time fixes the price of Opium, which is paid to cultivator.

C. REGARDING MANUFACTURE OF OPIUM

Only Central Government can manufacture opium at Government Opium Factory at Ghazipur and Memuch.

D. REGARDING SALEOF OPIUM

Sale of opium to State Government or manufacturing chemist can be made only from Government opium factory, Ghazipur.

E. EXPORT OF OPIUM:

The opium can be exported only on behalf of Central Government.

F. REGARDING MANUFACTURED DRUGS AND PYSCHOTROPIC SUBSTANCES

1.   The manufacture of crude Cocaine, ecognine and its salts and diacetylmorphine and its salt is prohibited.

2.   Cocaine hydrochloride can be manufactured by chemical staff of Government from confisticated cocaine.

3.   Morphine, Codeine, Thebaine and other alkaloids of opium can be manufactured only by Government Opium Factory.

4. Medicinal hemp can be manufactured under the condition of licence issued by the Narcotic Commissioner.

5. Psychotropic substance can be made in accordance with a licence under Drug and Cosmetic Act.

G. REGARDING IMPORT/EXPORT/TRANSHIPMENT OF NARCOTIC DRUGS/PSYCHOTROPIC SUBSTANCE

1. The import, export and transhipment of Coca leaf, Cannabis, Heroin are prohibited.

2. Only Government Opium Factory can import opium, concentrate of poppy straw, morphine, codeine, theabine and their salts.

3. Import of narcotic drug and psychotropic substances listed in schedule-II made only under licence.

4. Export of opium made only on behalf of Central Government.

5. Export of Narcotic Drugs and Psychotropic Substance listed in Schedule-II made only under licence.

6. The consignment of Narcotic Drug or Psychotropic Substance listed in Schedule-II can be transhipped at any port with permission of Custom Collector.

5.8 PROCEDURE

POWER TO ISSUE WARRANT AND AUTHORISATION

1. A Metropolitan Magistrate or a Magistrate of the first class or any Magistrate of the second class specially empowered by the State Government in this behalf, may issue a warrant for the arrest of any person whom he has reason to believe to have committed any offence punishable under Chapter IV, or for the search, whether by day or by night, of any building, conveyance or place in which he has reason to believe any narcotic drug or psychotropic substance in respect of which an offence punishable under Chapter IV has been committed or any document or other article which may furnish evidence of the commission of such offence is kept or concealed.

2. Any such officer of gazetted rank of the departments of central excise, narcotics, customs, revenue intelligence or any other department of the Central Government or of the Border Security Force as is empowered in this behalf by general or special order by the Central Government, or any such officer of the revenue, drugs control, excise, police or any other department of a State Government as is empowered in this behalf by general or special order of the State Government, if he has reason to believe from personal knowledge or information given by any person and taken in writing that any person has committed an offence punishable under Chapter IV or that any narcotic drug, or psychotropic substance in respect of which any offence punishable under Chapter IV has been committed or any document or other article which may furnish evidence of the commission of such offence has been kept or concealed in any building, conveyance or place, may authorise any officer subordinate to him but superior in rank to a peon, sepoy, or a constable, to arrest such a person or search a building, conveyance or place whether by day or by nigh or himself arrest a person or search a building, conveyance or place.

3. The officer to whom a warrant under sub-section (1) is addressed and the officer who authorised the arrest or search or the officer who is so authorised under sub-section (2) shall have all the powers of an officer acting under section 42.

POWER OF ENTRY, SEARCH, SEIZURE AND ARREST WITHOUT WARRANT OR AUTHORISATION

1. Any such officer (being an officer superior in rank to a peon, sepoy or constable) of the departments of central excise, narcotics, customs, revenue intelligence or any other department of the Central Government or of the Border Security Force as is embowered in this behalf by general or special order by the Central Government, or any such officer (being an officer superior in rank to a peon, sepoy or constable) of the revenue, drugs control, excise, police or any other department of a State Government as is empowered in this behalf by general or special

order of the State Government, if he has reason to believe from personal knowledge or information given by any person and taken down in writing, that any narcotic drug, or psychotropic substance, in respect of which an offence punishable under Chapter IV has been committed or any document or other article which may furnish evidence of the commission of such offence is kept or concealed in any building, conveyance or enclosed place, may, between sunrise and sunset –

a) enter into and search any such building, conveyance or place;

b) in case of resistance, break open any door and remove any obstacle to such entry;

c) seize such drug or substance and all materials used in the manufacture thereof and any other article and any animal or conveyance which he has reason to believe to be liable to confiscation under this Act and any document or other article which he has reason to believe may furnish evidence of the commission of any offence punishable under Chapter IV relating to such drug or substance:

Provided that if such officer has reason to believe that a search warrant or authorisation cannot be obtained without affording opportunity for the concealment of evidence or facility for the escape of an offender, he may enter and search such building, conveyance or enclosed place at any time between sunset and sunrise after recording the grounds of his belief.

2. Where an officer takes down any information in writing under sub-section (1) or records grounds for his belief under the proviso thereto, he shall forthwith send a copy thereof to his immediate official superior.

POWER OF SEIZURE AND ARREST IN PUBLIC PLACES

Any officer of any of the departments mentioned in section 42 may –

1. seize, in any public place or in transit, any narcotic drug or psychotropic substance in respect of which he has reason to

believe an offence punishable under Chapter IV has been committed, and, along with such drug or substance, any animal or conveyance or article liable to confiscation under this Act, and any document or other article which he has reason to believe may furnish evidence of the commission of an offence punishable under Chapter IV relating to such drug or substance;

2. detain and search any person whom he has reason to believe to have committed an offence punishable under Chapter IV, and, if such person has any narcotic drug or psychotropic substance in his possession and such possession appears to him to be unlawful, arrest him and any other person in his company.

POWER OF ENTRY, SEARCH, SEIZURE AND ARREST IN OFFENCES RELATING TO COCA PLANT, OPIUM POPPY AND CANNABIS PLANT

The provisions of sections 41, 42 and 43, shall so far as may be, apply in relation to the offence punishable under Chapter IV and relating to coca plant, the opium poppy or cannabis plant and for this purpose references in those sections to narcotic drugs, or psychotropic substance, shall be construed as including references to coca plant, the opium poppy and cannabis plant.

PROCEDURE WHERE SEIZURE OF GOODS LIABLE TO CONFISCATION NOT PRACTICABLE

Where it is not practicable to seize any goods (including standing crop) which are liable to confiscation under this Act, any officer duly authorised under section 42 may serve on the owner or person in possession of the goods, an order that he shall not remove, part with or otherwise deal with the goods except with the previous permission of such officer.

DUTY OF LAND HOLDER TO GIVE INFORMATION OF ILLEGAL CULTIVATION

very older of land shall give immediate information to any officer of the Police or of any of the departments mentioned in section 42 of all the opium poppy, cannabis plant or coca plant which may be illegally cultivated within his land and every such holder of and who knowingly neglects to give such information, shall be liable to punishment.

DUTY OF CERTAIN OFFICERS TO GIVE INFORMATION OF ILLEGAL CULTIVATION

Every officer of the Government and every panch, sarpanch and other village officer of whatever description shall give immediate information to any officer of the Police or of any of the departments mentioned in section 42 when it may come to his knowledge that any land has been illegally cultivated with the opium poppy, cannabis plant or coca plant, and every such officer of the Government, panch, sarpanch and other village officer who neglects to give such information shall be liable to punishment.

POWER OF ATTACHMENT OF CROP ILLEGALLY CULTIVATED

Any Metropolitan Magistrate, Judicial Magistrate of the first class or any Magistrate specially empowered in this behalf by the State Government [or any officer of a gazetted rank empowered under section 42] may order attachment of any opium poppy, cannabis plant or coca plant which he has reason to believe to have been illegally cultivated and while doing so may pass such order (including an order to destroy the crop) as he thinks fit.

POWER TO STOP AND SEARCH CONVEYANCE

Any officer authorised under section 42, may, if he has reason to suspect that any animal or conveyance is, or is about to be, used for the transport of any narcotic drug or psychotropic substance, in respect of which he suspects that any provision of this Act has been, or is being, or is about to be, contravened at any time, stop such animal or conveyance, or, in the case of an aircraft, compel it to land and –

1. rummage and search the conveyance or part thereof;
2. examine and search any goods on the animal or in the conveyance;

3.   if it becomes necessary to stop the animal or the conveyance, he may use all lawful means for stopping it, and where such means fail, the animal or the conveyance may be fired upon.

CONDITIONS UNDER WHICH SEARCH OF PERSONS SHALL BE CONDUCTED

1.   When any officer duly authorised under section 42 is about to search any person under the provisions of section 41, section 42 or section 43, he shall, if such person so requires, take such person without unnecessary delay to nearest Gazetted Officer of any of the departments mentioned in section 42 or to the nearest Magistrate.

2.   If such requisition is made, the officer may detain the person until he can bring him before the Gazetted Officer or the Magistrate referred to in sub-section (1).

3.   The Gazetted Officer or the Magistrate before whom any such person is brought shall, if he sees no reasonable ground for search, forthwith discharge the person but otherwise shall direct that search be made.

4.   No female shall be searched by anyone excepting a female.

PROVISIONS OF THE CODE OF CRIMINAL PROCEDURE, 1973 TO APPLY TO WARRANTS, ARRESTS, SEARCHES AND SEIZURES

The provisions of the Code of Criminal Procedure, 1973 (2 of 1974) shall apply, in so far as they are not inconsistent with the provisions of this Act, to all warrants issued and arrests, searches and seizures made under this Act.

DISPOSAL OF PERSONS ARRESTED AND ARTICLES SEIZED

1.   Any officer arresting a person under section 41, section 42, section 43 or section 44 shall, as soon as may be, inform him of the grounds for such arrest.

2.   Every person arrested and article seized under warrant issued under sub-section (1) of section 41 shall be forwarded without

unnecessary delay to the Magistrate by whom the warrant was issued.

OFFENCES AND PENALTIES

S.NO	OFFENCES	PENALTIES
1.	a) Contravention of provision in respect of- Poppy straw, Opium poppy, Coca plant, Coca leaves, Prepared Opium, Manufactured drug, Psychotropic substances. b) Illegal import or export or external dealing if narcotic drugs or psychotropic substance. c) Allowing the use of premises, vehicle etc for commission of an offence. d) Misappropriation of opium by licensed cultivators. e) Contravention in respect of cannabis and cannabis other than ganja.	a) 10-25 years imprisonment and fine of 1 lacs – 2 lacs, in case of first conviction. b) 15-30 years imprisonment and fine of 1.5 lacs– 3 lacs, in case of subsequent conviction.
2.	Contravention with respect to cannabis and ganja.	a) 5 years imprisonment and fine up to Rs 50,000/-, in case of first conviction. b) 10 years imprisonment and fine up to Rs 1,00,000/-, in case of subsequent conviction.

Continued on next page

S.NO	OFFENCES	PENALTIES
3.	Failure to keep account, false account, false statement, failure to produce licence, indulgence in a breach of any provision of the Act.	a) 5 years imprisonment or fine or both. b) 10 years imprisonment or fine or both.
4.	Illegal possession for personal consumption of cocaine, morphine or other narcotic drugs or psychotropic substances.	1 year imprisonment or fine or both.
5.	Illegal possession for personal consumption other than those specified in (4) above.	6 months imprisonment or fine or both.

REVIEW QUESTIONS

ESSAY QUESTIONS

1. Write a note on administrative committees under the narcotic drugs and psychotropic substance act 1985.

2. Write a note on power of Central Government to Permit, Control and Regulate the operations regarding the Narcotic Drugs and Psychotropic Substances.

3. Write a note on power of State Government to Permit, Control and Regulate the operations regarding the Narcotic Drugs and Psychotropic Substances.

SHORT QUESTIONS

1. What are the objectives of Narcotic drugs and Psychotropic substances Act 1985?

2. Define.

   a) Cannabis.

   b) Coca derivative.

   c) Controlled substances.

   d) Illicit traffic.

3. Write a note on special provisions regarding Cultivation, Production and Export of Opium.

4. Write a note on various Offences and Penalties under the Narcotic drugs and Psychotropic substance Act 1985.

MCQ's

1. The Narcotic drugs and Psychotropic substance Act was passed in,

   a) 1958

   b) 1895

   c) 1985

   d) 1965.

2. The Narcotic drugs and Psychotropic substance Advisory committee is also called as.

   a) Executive committee.

   b) Consultative committee.

   c) Administrative committee.

   d) Both (b) and (c).

3. The Narcotic drugs and Psychotropic substance Advisory committee consist of how many members (except the chairman)?

   a) 25

   b) 25 +

   c) 20 +

   d) 20.

4. The officers of Narcotic drugs and Psychotropic substances Executive committee are appointed by,

   a) State government.

   b) Central government.

   c) Both (a) and (b).

   d) None of the above.

5. The licence for the cultivation of Opium poppy is granted by,

   a) Narcotic commissioner.

   b) State Opium Officer.

   c) District opium officer.

   d) Lambardar.

6. Opium can be manufacture only by,

   a) Lambardar.

   b) Government opium factory.

   c) Both (a) and (b).

   d) None of the above.

7. Export of opium is done only by.

   a) State government.

   b) Central government.

   c) Both (a) and (b).

   d) None of the above.

8. The licence for the manufacture of Medicinal Hemp is granted by,

   a) Central government.

   b) State government.

   c) Narcotic commissioner.

   d) None of the above.

9. The licence for the manufacture of Narcotic substance is granted by,

   a) State government.

   b) Central government.

   c) Narcotic commissioner.

   d) None of the above.

10. The price of opium is fixed by,

    a) Executive committee.

    b) State government.

    c) Central government.

    d) None of the above.

ANSWERS: 1-c, 2-d, 3-d, 4-c, 5-c, 6-b, 7-b, 8-b, 9-c, 10-c.

Chapter 6

DRUG (PRICE CONTROL) ORDER 1995

6.1 INTRODUCTION

This order was made under section 3 of essential commodities Act, 1955. The first act pertaining to price control termed as "drug price (display and control) order" was passed in 1966 and then amended as follows:

- Drug (price control) order, 1970
- Drug (price control) order, 1979
- Drug (price control) order, 1987
- Drug (price control) order, 1995

OBJECTIVES

Drug (price control) order wad amended in order to meet the following objectives.

1. To ensure equitable distribution of essential bulk drugs.

2. To fix the maximum retail price for drug formulation in order to meet profit.

3. To exercise government control over the price of bulk drug and drug formulation.

DEFINITIONS

1. ***Bulk drug:*** A substance either pharmaceutical, chemical, biological or plant product and/or its salt, esters, sterio-isomers

and derivatives conforming to pharmacopoeial or other standards accepted under the Drug and Cosmetic Act-1940 which is used as such or as an ingredient in any formulation.

2. *Formulation:* A pharmaceutical product containing one or more bulk drug(s) with or without the use of any pharmaceutical aids meant for internal or external use.

3. *Local taxes:* It is any tax or levy paid to the central or state government or any local authority under any law by the manufacturer.

4. *Retailer:* A dealer carrying on the retail business of sale of drugs to customer.

5. *Ceiling price:* Net price fixed by the government for scheduled formulation keeping in view the cost or efficiency or both of major manufacturer of such formulations.

6. *Retail price:* Price of the drug fixed in accordance with the provision of this order and includes ceiling price.

7. *Wholesaler:* A stockist or his agent appointed by a manufacturer or an importer for the sale of his drugs to retailer, hospital, dispensary, medical, educational or research institution purchasing bulk quantities of drugs.

8. *Scheduled bulk drug:* A bulk drug specified in the first schedule.

9. *Non-scheduled bulk drug:* A bulk drug not specified in first schedule.

10. *Scheduled formulation:* A formulation containing any bulk drug specified in the first schedule either individually or in combination with other drug or drugs not specified in the first schedule except single ingredient formulation based on bulk drugs specified in the first schedule or sold under the generic name.

11. *Non-scheduled formulation:* A formulation not containing any bulk drugs specified in the first schedule.

6.2 PROVISIONS OF THE ACT

The various provisions of the act are as follows,

1. Fix prices of bulk drugs in first scheduled.

2. Fix retail prices of formulation.

3. Fix prices to wholesaler and retailer.

4. Schedules.

6.3 PRICES OF BULK DRUGS IN FIRST SCHEDULED

In order to fix the maximum sale price of bulk drug, Central Government established National Pharmaceutical Pricing Authority (NPPA) in August 1997. Prices are fixed after proper enquiry and for this purpose of enquiry, details in form I and additional details are furnished by the manufacturer twice a year.

In fixing price of a bulk drug government considers the following things.

1. A post tax return of 14% on net worth (18% if production is from basic stage) OR

2. A return of 22% on capital employed(26% if production is from basic stage) OR

3. Internal rate return of 12% based on long term marginal costing for a new plant.

Manufacturer may exercise any option of returns. For any change in rate of returns approval from the government is needed.

A bulk drug should be sold at the fixed prices plus local taxes if any, not at a higher price.

Any manufacturer who wishes to manufacture bulk drug or existing manufacturer wishes to manufacture additional bulk drug then they have to give all necessary details within 15days of commencement of production so that government can notify its price.

Any manufacturer who desirers revision of the maximum sale price of a bulk drug fixed, shall make an application to the government in form I, after making enquiry, government will fix a revised price (within 4 months).

No manufacturer or distributor can refuse sale of bulk drug any other dealer. The government can direct any manufacturer of bulk drug to sell the same to formulators.

6.4 RETAIL PRICES OF FORMULATION

National Pharmaceutical Pricing Authority (NPPA) is also responsible for fixing the retail price of formulation. It is calculated as follows.

$$R.P = [M.C + C.C + P.M + P.C] [1+ M.U / 100]$$

(as per order 1979)

$$R.P = [M.C + C.C + P.M + P.C] [1+ M.A.P.E / 100] + E.D$$

(as per order 1987 and 1995)

Where,

R.P = retail price.

M.C = material cost (drug + pharmaceutical aids + overages + process loss).

C.C = conversion cost.

P.M = packing material cost.

P.C = packing charges.

M.U = mark up (manufacturer's margin + promotional expenses + outward freight + distribution cost + trade commission.)

M.A.P.E = maximum allowable post manufacturing expenses (all cost incurred by a manufacturer from the stage of ex-factory cost to r   etailing and include trade margin.)

E.D = excise duty.

The different categories of formulation as per DPCO 1991 are,

- Category I formulations- Formulations contains any bulk drug either individually or in combination specified for Category I formulations.

- Category II- Formulations contains any bulk drug either individually or in combination specified for Category II formulations.

- If formulation contains bulk drugs specified in both Category I and II then it is considered to be Category I formula.

Different values of M.A.P.E (M.U) are fixed for different categories of formulation as per DPCO 1991 as follows,

- 75% in the case of Category I formulation of the third schedule.

- 100% in the case of Category II formulation of the third schedule.

- 100% in the case of formulation indigenously Manufactured Scheduled formulation.

6.5 PRICE TO WHOLESALER AND RETAILER

For a scheduled product, the prices of purchase for a wholesaler and retailer are as follows,

- Wholesaler purchase price = R.P − 20%

- Retailer purchase price = R.P − 16%

SCHEDULES

There are three schedules to this Act,

1. Schedule I: List of bulk drugs (76) used in scheduled formulations.

2. Schedule II: List of forms.

3. Schedule III: Comprise pre-tax return on sale turn-over of formulation of different category of unit.

6.6 SCHEDULE I

(List of bulk drug used in Scheduled formulation)

S.No	Name of Drugs	S.No	Name of Drugs
1.	Sulphamethoxazole	39.	Griseofulvin
2.	Penicillins	40.	Gentamicin
3.	Tetracycline	41.	Dextropropoxyphene
4.	Rifampicin	42.	Halogenated hydroxyquinoline
5.	Streptomycin	43.	Pentazocine
6.	Ranitidine	44.	Captopril
7.	Vitamin C	45.	Naproxen
8.	Betamethasone	46.	Pyrental
9.	Metronidazole	47.	Sulphadoxine
10.	Chloroquine	48.	norfloxacin
11.	Insulin	49.	Cefadroxyl
12.	Erythromycin	50.	Panthonates & panthenols
13.	Vitamin A	51.	Furazolidone
14.	Oxytetracyclsine	52.	Pyrithioxine
15.	Prednisole	53.	Sulphadiazine
16.	Cephazolin	54.	Framycetin
17.	Methyldopa	55.	Verapamil
18.	Aspirin	56.	Amikacin sulphate
19.	Trimethoprin	57.	Glipizide
20.	Cloxacillin	58.	Spironolactone
21.	Sulphadimidine	59.	Pentoxyfyline
22.	Salbutamol	60.	Amodiaquin
23.	Famotidine	61.	Sulphamoxole
24.	Ibuprofen	62.	Frusemide
25.	Analgin	63.	Pheniramine maleate
26.	Doxycycline	64.	Chloroxylenols
27.	Ciprofloxacin	65.	Becampicillin
28.	Cefotaxime	66.	Lincomycin
29.	Dexamethasone	67.	Chloropropamide

Continued on next page

S.No	Name of Drugs	S.No	Name of Drugs
30.	Ephedrine	68.	Mebhydroline
31.	Vitamin B1	69.	Chloropromazine
32.	Carbamazepine	70.	Methendienone
33.	Vitamin B2	71.	Phenyl butazone
34.	Theophylline	72.	Lynestranol
35.	Levodopa	73.	Salazosulphapyrine
36.	Tolnaftate	74.	Diosmine
37.	Vitamin E	75.	Trimipramine
38.	Nalidixic acid	76.	Mefenamic acid

REVIEW QUESTIONS

1. Define.

   a) Bulk drug.

   b) Formulation.

   c) Scheduled formulation.

   d) Wholesaler.

2. Write the Objectives and the Provision of Drug (Price Control) Order 1995.

3. How are the prices for the Bulk drug in first schedule fixed?

4. Write and explain the formula used to calculate the Retail price of Formulation.

MCQ's

1. In August 1997, which authority did the central government establish in order to enquire and fix the price for the bulk drug?

   a) National Pharmaceutical Packing Authority.

   b) National Pharmaceutical Pricing Authority.

   c) National Pharmaceutical Purchasing Authority.

   d) National Pharmaceutical Processing Authority.

2. For the purpose of enquiry the details in form I are furnished by the manufacturer,

   a) Once in six months.

   b) Once in a year.

   c) Once in two years.

   d) Twice a month.

3. In fixing price of a bulk drug government considers the following things.

   a)   A post tax return of 14% on net worth (18% if production is from basic stage)

   b)   A return of 22% on capital employed(26% if production is from basic stage)

   c)   Internal rate return of 12% based on long term marginal costing for a new plant.

   d) Any one of the above three.

4. M.A.P.E

   a)   Minimum allowable packing expenses.

   b)   Minimum allowable purchasing expenses.

   c)   Maximum allowable post-manufacturing expenses.

   d)   Maximum allowable pre-manufacturing expenses.

5. For a scheduled formulation, the manufacturer selling price is,

   a)   R.P – 20%

   b)   R.P – 16%

   c)   R.P – 12%

   d)   R.P – 10%

Answers: 1-b, 2-a, 3-d, 4-c, 5-a

Chapter 7

DRUGS AND MAGIC REMEDIES (OBJECTIONAL ADVERTISEMENTS) ACT 1954 AND RULE 1955

7.1 INTRODUCTION

The Act was passed on 1st April, 1955 and was amended in 1963. An Act to control the advertisement of drugs in certain cases, to prohibit the advertisement for certain purposes of remedies alleged to possess magic qualities and to provide for matters connected therewith.

This Act may be called the Drugs and Magic Remedies (Objectionable Advertisements) Act, 1954.

It extends to the whole of India except the State of Jammu and Kashmir, and applies also to persons domiciled in the territories to which this Act extends who are outside the said territories.

It shall come into force on such date as the Central Government may, by notification in the Official Gazette, appoint.

OBJECTIVES

1. To control the advertisement of drugs.

2. To prohibit the advertisement for certain purposes of Remedies alleged to possess magic qualities.

DEFINITIONS

1. *Advertisement:* It includes any notice, circular, label, wrapper, or other document, and any announcement made orally or by any means of producing or transmitting light, sound or smoke.

2.   ***Magic remedy:*** It includes a talisman, mantra, kavacha, and any other charm of any kind which is alleged to possess miraculous powers for or in the diagnosis, cure, mitigation, treatment or prevention of any disease in human beings or animals or for affecting or influencing in any way the structure or any organic function of the body of human beings or animals.

3.   ***Venereal diseases:*** It includes Syphilis, Gonorrhea, Soft chancre, venereal granuloma and Lymphogranuloma.

7.2 PROHIBITION OF ADVERTISEMENT OF CERTAIN DRUGS FOR TREATMENT OF CERTAIN DISEASES AND DISORDERS

Subject to the provisions of this Act, no person shall take any part in the publication of any advertisement referring to any drug in terms which suggest or are calculated to lead to the use of that drug for,

a)   The procurement of miscarriage in women or prevention of conception in women; or

b)   The maintenance or improvement of the capacity of human beings for sexual pleasure; or

c)   The correction of menstrual disorder in women; or

d)   The diagnosis, cure, mitigation, treatment or prevention of any disease, disorder or condition specified in the Schedule J, or any other disease, disorder or condition which may be specified in the rules made under this Act.

Provided that no such rule shall be made except,

a)   In respect of any disease, disorder or condition which requires timely treatment in consultation with a registered medical practitioner or for which there are normally no accepted remedies, and

b)   after consultation with the Drugs Technical Advisory Board constituted under the Drugs and Cosmetics Act, 1940 and, if the

Central Government considers necessary, with such other persons having special knowledge or practical experience in respect of Ayurvedic or Unani systems of medicines as that Government deems fit.

7.3 PROHIBITION OF MISLEADING ADVERTISEMENTS RELATING TO DRUGS

Subject to the provisions of this Act, no person shall take any part in the publication of any advertisement relating to a drug if the advertisement contains any matter which,

a) Directly or indirectly gives a false impression regarding the true character of the drug; or

b) Makes a false claim for the drug; or

c) Is otherwise false or misleading in any material particular.

7.4 PROHIBITION OF ADVERTISEMENT OF MAGIC REMEDIES FOR TREATMENT OF CERTAIN DISEASES AND DISORDERS

No person carrying on or purporting to carry on the profession of administering magic remedies shall take any part in the publication of any advertisement referring to any magic remedy which directly or indirectly claims to be efficacious for any of the purposes specified in section 3.

7.5 PROHIBITION OF ADVERTISEMENT OF DRUG

Any drugs with following conditions are prohibited from advertisement.

1. Contains statements which are considered to be offensive to good taste or are misleading.

2. Designed to arouse unwarranted expectation of product effectiveness.

3. Misleading with regard to its safety, usage or immediacy of relief.

4. Derogatory to other competing products.

5. Allows statements which create fear or apprehension in the public mind such as a person may suffer from an ailment by not using a particular product.

6. Allows offer of rewards or other inducement leading to excessive use of drug by a consumer.

7. Gives an impression that a medical consultation or surgical operation is unnecessary.

8. Refers to or implies reference to the statutory bodies like Drug Control Authorities, Medical council, Dental Council, Government Laboratories etc.

9. Includes products which are required to be sold only against prescriptions written by registered medical practitioner.

10. Contains a claim which makes reference either directly or indirectly or by implication to the diseases mentioned in the Schedule J of drug and magic remedies (objectionable advertisements) Act 1954 and rules made thereunder.

11. Make any claim or statement that it is universal panacea, infallible, unfailing, miraculous, a certainty, guaranteed or sure cure.

12. Imply that it is recommended by health professionals i.e. Medical practitioner, Psychologist, Dentist, Nurses, Pharmacists, Practitioners of Ayurvedic, Siddha, Unani or Homeopathic system of medicine, unless scientifically substantiated.

13. Advertisement for non prescription systemic analgesic shall carry warning "use only as directed ". This must be clear visible or audible or legible.

14. An advertisement for Vitamins preparation and Tonics shall not infer that such products are a substitute for good nutrition or could replace a balanced diet.

7.6   PROHIBITION OF IMPORT INTO, AND EXPORT FROM, INDIA OF CERTAIN ADVERTISEMENTS

No person shall import into, or export from, the territories to which this Act extends any document containing an advertisement of the nature referred to in section 3, or section 4, or section 5, and any documents containing any such advertisement shall be deemed to be goods of which the import or export has been prohibited under section 19 of the Sea Customs Act, 1878 and all the provisions of that Act shall have effect accordingly, except that section 183 thereof shall have effect as if for the word 'shall' therein the word 'may' were substituted.

7.7 EXEMPTED ADVERTISEMENTS

The following classes of advertisements are exempted from the provision of prohibition.

1. Any sign board or notice displayed by a Registered Medical Practitioner on his premises indicating that treatment is under taken for any disease, disorder or condition.

2. Books or Treatises dealing with the diseases published from bonifide scientific or social standpoint.

3. Advertisement relating to drugs which are sent confidentially to R.M.P, it should bear the following words on top "For the use of R.M.P only".

4. Any advertisement relating to drug printed or published by the government.

5. Any advertisement relating to drug printed or published by any person with previous permission of government.

6. Labels or set of instructions sent with package of product which is permitted under Drug and Cosmetic Act.

7.8 EXEMPTED ADVERTISEMENTS WITH CONDITIONS (notification issued in 1967)

The following classes of advertisements are also exempted from the provision of prohibition under some conditions.

1. Leaflets or literature sent with packaging or advertisement of drugs in medical, pharmaceutical scientific technical journal.

   Condition: advertisement should contain only such information which are required for guidance of R.M.P such as Therapeutic indication, Route of administration, Dose, Side effects, Precautions etc.

2. Price list or Therapeutic index published by Manufacturer, Importer or Medical literature distributed by Medical representatives.

   Condition: It should contain only such information which are required for the guidance of R.M.P such as Therapeutic indication, Route of administration, Dose, Side effects, Precautions etc. The distribution of such literature is limited to R.M.P, Hospital, Dispensary, Medical and Research Institutes.

7.9 CODE OF ETHICS FOR ADVERTISEMENT OF DRUGS

Model guidelines

The text document finalised by subcommittee on Code of Ethics for Advertisement of Drugs under the Directorate General of Health Service and as received from Drug controller of India is reproduced here.

Code for advertising drugs in India (Preamble)

1. Objective of this code – to ensure responsible advertisement of drugs (or medicine) in promoting their sale which may be purchased by the public without prescription and for which therapeutic claims are made.

2. The following have to be considered while evolving the code,

a) World Health Organisation "Ethical Criteria for medicinal drug Promotion 1988", in particular "Advertisements in all form to the general public".

b) Advertisement ethics and code of Medical Standards of Indian Newspaper Society as appearing in its publication- "Rules governing accreditation of Advertising laid down by Prasar Bharti".

c) Code for commercial advertisements laid down by Prasar Bharti.

d) Drugs and Magic remedies (Objectionable Advertisement) Act 1954 and Rules made thereunder,

e) Guidelines for Voluntary Codes of advertising practices- laid by world federation of Proprietary Medicines Manufactures.

f) Organisation of Pharmaceuticals Producers of India (OPP) guidelines on "IFPMA Code on Pharmaceutical Marketing Practices".

g) Indian Drug Manufacturer's Association (IDMA) guidelines on "Pharmaceutical Marketing Practices".

Self-medication is an important element in health care. Thus advertisement of medicinal products to general public needs to satisfy certain criteria. Advertisement is an important promotional tool, it also serves public legitimate desire of information concerned to their health and helps public to make rational decisions on the use of medicines which are legally available without prescriptions (over the counter, OTC) drugs. This code in any way does not imply that advertisers are restricted in using advertising media as a means of Education and dissemination of information to public in general.

The primary source of information about the product is the pharmaceutical industry. These industries have the responsibility to ensure that medicinal products belonging to any system of medicine are advertised in a responsible manner conforming to the principles set out in this code. The industry association as well as individual pharmaceutical manufacturing/marketing firms are advised to adopt the guidelines set out in this code for the commercial advertising of their products.

This code forms the core component of the ethical guidelines, which may be formulated by individual industry association and the media etc.

7.10 OFFENCES AND PENALTIES

Offences: Anyone who contravenes any provision of this Act by taking part in prohibition advertisement.

Penalties: Six months imprisonment or fine or both on first conviction.

One year imprisonment or fine or both on any subsequent conviction.

POWERS OF ENTRY AND SEARCH

1.   Subject to the provisions of any rules made in this behalf, any Gazetted Officer authorised by the State Government may, within the local limits of the area for which he is so authorized,

a)   Enter and search at all reasonable times, with such assistants, if any, as he considers necessary, any place in which he has reason to believe that an offence under this Act has been or is being committed.

b)   Seize any advertisement which he has reason to believe contravenes any of the provisions of this Act.

Provided that the power of seizure under this clause may be exercised in respect of any document, article or thing which contains any such advertisement, including the contents, if any, of such document, article or thing, if the advertisement cannot be separated by reason of its being embossed or otherwise, from such document, article or thing without affecting the integrity, utility or saleable value thereof.

c)   Examine any record, register, document or any other material object found in any place mentioned in clause (a) and seize the same if he has reason to believe that it may furnish evidence of the commission of an offence punishable under this Act.

2. The provisions of the Code of Criminal Procedure, 1898 (5 of 1898) shall, so far as may be, apply to any search or seizure under this Act as they apply to any search or seizure made under the authority of a warrant issued under section 98 of the said Code.

3. Where any person seizes anything under clause (b) or clause (c) of sub-section (1), he shall, as soon as may be, inform a Magistrate and take his orders as to the custody thereof.

OFFENCES BY COMPANIES

1. If the person contravening any of the provisions of this Act is a company, every person who, at the time the offence was committed, was in charge of, and was responsible to, the company for the conduct of the business of the company as well as the company shall be deemed to be guilty of the contravention and shall be liable to be proceeded against and punished accordingly:

   Provided that nothing contained in this sub-section shall render any such person liable to any punishment provided in this Act if he proves that the offence was committed without his knowledge or that he exercised all due diligence to prevent the commission of such offence.

2. Notwithstanding anything contained in sub-section (1) where an offence under this Act has been committed by a company and it is proved that the offence was committed with the consent or connivance of, or is attributable to any neglect on the part of, any director or manager, secretary or the officer of the company, such director, manager, secretary or other officer of the company shall also be deemed to be guilty of that offence and shall be liable to be proceeded against and punished accordingly.

7.11 POWER TO EXEMPT FROM APPLICATION OF ACT

If in the opinion of the Central Government public interest requires that the advertisement of any specified drug or class of drugs or any specified class of advertisements relating to drugs, should be permitted, it may, by notification in the Official Gazette, direct that the provisions of sections 3, 4, 5 and 6 or any one of such provisions shall not apply or shall apply subject to such conditions as may be specified in the notification to or in relation to the advertisement of any such drug or class of drugs [or any such class of advertisements relating to drugs.

POWER TO MAKE RULES

1. The Central Government may, by notification in the Official Gazette, make rules for carrying out the purposes of this Act.

2. In particular and without prejudice to the generality of the foregoing power, such rules may.

a) Specify any disease, disorder or condition to which the provisions of section 3 shall apply.

b) Prescribe the manner in v.hich advertisements of articles or things referred to in clause (c) of section 14 may be sent confidentially.

3. Every rule made under this Act shall be laid, as soon as may be after it is made, before each of House of Parliament while it is in session for a total period of thirty days which be comprised in one session or in two or more successive sessions and if before the expiry of the session in which it is so laid or the successive sessions aforesaid, both Houses agree in making any modification in the rule or both Houses agree that the rule should not be made, the rule shall thereafter have effect only in such modified form or be of no effect, as the case may be; so however, that any such modification or annulment shall be without prejudice to the validity of anything previously done under that rule.

7.12 SCHEDULE TO THE ACT

There is Schedule J which comprises list of Diseases/Conditions which are incurable and a Drug may not purport to Prevent or Cure or Make Claims to Prevent or Cure such diseases/conditions.

The list of such diseases/condition is given below (SCHEDULE 'J').

Appendicitis.	Hydrocele
Arteriosclerosis.	Hysteria
Blindness.	Infantile paralysis
Blood poisoning	Insanity
Bright's disease	Leprosy
Cancer	Leucoderma
Cataract	Lockjaw
Deafness	Locomotor ataxia
Diabetes.	Lupus
Diseases and Disorders of brain.	Nervous debility
Diseases and Disorders of the optical system.	Obesity
	Plague
Diseases and Disorders of the uterus.	Pleurisy
	Pneumonia
Disorders of menstrual flow.	Rheumatism
Disorders of the nervous system.	Ruptures
	Sexual impotence
Disorders of the prostatic gland.	Smallpox
Dropsy.	Stature of persons
Epilepsy.	Sterility in women
Female diseases (in general).	Trachoma
Fevers (in general).	Tuberculosis
Fits.	Typhoid fever
Form and structure of the female bust.	Ulcers of the gastro intestinal tract
	Venereal diseases Including
Gall stones kidney stones and bladder stones	syphilis, gonorrhoea, soft chancre, venereal granuloma and lympho
Gangrene.	granuloma
Glaucoma	Heart diseases
Goitre	Paralysis
High/Low Blood Pressure	
Tumours	

7.13   THE DRUGS AND MAGIC REMEDIES (OBJECTIONABLE ADVERTISEMENTS) RULES, 1955

INTRODUCTION

In exercise of the powers conferred by section 16 of the Drugs and Magic Remedies (Objectionable Advertisements) Act, 1954 (21 of 1954), the Central Government hereby makes the rules.

These rules may be called as the Drugs and Magic Remedies (Objectionable Advertisements) Rules, 1955.

They shall come into force on such date as the Central Government may, by notification in the Official Gazette, appoint.

SCRUTINY OF MISLEADING ADVERTISEMENTS RELATING TO DRUGS

Any person authorized by the State Government in this behalf may, if satisfied, that an advertisement relating to a drug contravenes the provisions of section 4, by order, require the manufacturer, packer, distributor or seller of the drug to furnish, within such time as may be specified in the order or such further time as may be allowed in this behalf by the person so authorized information regarding the composition of the drug or the ingredients thereof or any other information in regard to that drug as he deems necessary for holding the scrutiny of the advertisement and where any such order is made, it shall be the duty of the manufacturer, packer, distributor or seller of the drug to which the advertisement relates to comply with the order. Any failure to comply with such order shall, for the purposes of section 7, be deemed to be a contravention of the provisions of section 4.

Provided that no publisher or advertising agency of any medium for the dissemination of any advertisement relating to a drug shall be deemed to have made any contravention merely by reason of the dissemination by him or if any such advertisement, unless such publisher or advertising agency has failed to comply with any discretion made by the authorized person in this behalf calling upon him or it to furnish the name and address of the manufacturer, packer, distributor, seller or advertising agency, as the case may be, who or which caused such advertisement to be disseminated.

7.14 PROCEDURE TO BE FOLLOWED IN PROHIBITING IMPORT INTO, AND EXPORT FROM INDIA OF CERTAIN ADVERTISEMENTS

1. If the Customs Collector has reasons to believe that any consignment contains documents of the nature referred to in section 6, he may and if requested by an officer appointed for the purpose by the Central Government, shall detain the consignment and dispose it of in accordance with the provisions of the Sea Customs Act, 1878 , and the rules made thereunder, and shall also inform the importer or exporter of the order so passed.

   Provided that if the importer or exporter feels aggrieve by an order passed by the Customs Collector under this sub-rule and makes a representation to him within one week of the date of the order and has given an undertaking in writing not to dispose of the consignment without the consent of the Customs Collector and to return the consignment when so required to do by the Customs Collector, the Customs Collector shall pass an order making over the consignment to the importer or exporter, as the case may be/

   Provided further that before passing any order under this sub-rule or under the first proviso thereto, the Customs Collector shall consult the officer appointed for the purpose by Central Government.

2. If the importer or exporter who has given an undertaking under the first provision to sub rule (1) is required by the Customs Collector to return the consignment or any portion thereof, he shall return the consignment or portion thereof within ten days of the receipt of the notice.

MANNER IN WHICH ADVERTISEMENTS MAY BE SENT CONFIDENTIALLY

All documents containing advertisements relating to drugs referred to in clause (c) of sub-section (1) of section 14, shall be sent by post to a registered medical practitioner by name or to a wholesale or retail chemist, the address of such registered medical practitioner or wholesale or retail chemist being given. Such document shall bear at the top, printed in indelible ink in a conspicuous manner, the words. "For the use only of registered medical practitioners or a hospital or a laboratory"

7.15   PROHIBITION OF ADVERTISEMENT OF DRUGS FOR TREATMENT OF DISEASE

No person shall also take part in the publication of any advertisement referring to any drug in terms which suggest or are calculated to lead to the use of that drug for the diagnosis, cure, mitigation, treatment or prevention of any disease, disorder, or condition specified in the Schedule annexed to these rules.

REVIEW QUESTIONS

1. Write the objective of drugs and magic remedies act 1955 and define the following.

    a)   Advertisements.

    b)   Magic remedies.

    c)   Venereal disease.

2. What are the classes of advertisement prohibited to be advertised in Drugs and Magic remedies Act 1955?

3. What are the classes of drugs prohibited to be advertised in Drugs and Magic remedies Act 1955?

4. Write a note on procedure to be followed in prohibiting import into, and export from India of certain advertisements.

5. Write a note on advertisement exempted from the provision of Drugs and Magic remedies act 1955.

6. Write a note on advertisement exempted with conditions from the provision of Drugs and Magic remedies act 1955.

MCQ's

1. What is the main objective of Drug and Magic Remedies Act 1954?
    a) To control marketing of the drugs.
    b) To control the advertisement of the drugs.
    c) Both (a) and (b).
    d) None of the above.

2. What does the abbreviation OTC mean?
    a) Off the counter.
    b) Over the counter.
    c) Over the cash.
    d) Outside the country.

3. Which of the following is not a prohibited advertisement?
    a) Advertisement claiming to correct menstrual disorders in women.
    b) Advertisement relating to claim efficacy for Schedule J diseases.
    c) Advertisement relating to drugs sent confidentially to R.M.P.
    d) None of the above.

4. The Rules for Drug and Magic Remedies Act was passed in?
    a) 1945.
    b) 1954.
    c) 1955.
    d) 1965.

Answers: 1-b, 2-b, 3-c, 4-c

Chapter 8

IMPORTANT ACTS

PART A

PREVENTION OF CRUELTY TO ANIMALS ACT, 1960

8.1 INTRODUCTION

1. This Act may be called the Prevention of Cruelty to Animals Act, 1960.

2. It extends to the whole of India except the State of Jammu and Kashmir.

3. It shall come into force on such date as the Central Government may, by notification in the official Gazette, appoint, and different dates may be appointed for different States and for the different provisions contained in this Act.

OBJECTIVES

In modern medical and pharmaceutical sciences, animals are widely used to perform experiments to study the safety, toxicity and therapeutic efficacy of drugs as they are much similar to human systems.

Animals may be subjected to injury, pain or suffering and even death. The Act prevents the infliction of unnecessary pain or suffering on animals. The Act prevents the human from behaving cruel toward animals.

DEFINITION

1. *Animal:* Means any living creature other than a human being.

2. *Captive animal:* Means any animal (not being a domestic animal) which is in capacity or confinement, whether permanent or temporary, or which is subjected to any appliance of contrivance for the purpose of hindering or preventing its escape from captivity or confinement or which is pinioned or which is or appears to be maimed.

3. *Domestic animal:* Means any animal which is tamed or which has been or is being sufficiently tamed to serve some purpose for the use of man or which, although it neither has been nor is intended to be so tamed, is or has become in fact wholly or partly tamed.

4. *Local authority:* Means a municipal committee, district board or other authority for the time being invested by law with the control and administration of any matters within a specified local area.

5. *Cruelty:* Infliction of unnecessary pain or suffering.

6. *Breeder:* Mean a person including an institution, which breeds animal for the purpose of transfer to other authorised institution for performing experiments.

7. *Establishment:* Means any individual, company, firms, corporation, and institution other than school up to higher secondary level, which performs experiments on animals.

8. *Experiments:* Means any programme/project involving experiments on animals for the purpose of advancement by new discovery of physiological knowledge which will be for saving or prolonging life or alleviating suffering or for combating any disease whether on human being or animals.

8.2 ESTABLISHMENT OF ANIMAL WELFARE BOARD OF INDIA

1. For the promotion of animal welfare generally and for the purpose of protecting animals from being subjected to unnecessary pain or suffering, in particular, there shall be established by the Central

Government, as soon as may be after the commencement of this Act, a Board to be called the (Animal Board of India.)

2.   The Board shall be a body corporate having perpetual succession and a common seal with power, subject to the provisions of this Act, to acquire, hold and dispose of property and may by its name sue and is sued.

CONSTITUTION OF THE BOARD

1.   The Board shall consist of the following persons, namely:

(a) The Inspector General of Forests, Government of India, ex-officio.

(b) The Animal Husbandry Commissioner to the Government of India, ex-officio.

• Two persons to represent respectively the Ministries of the Central Government dealing with Home Affairs and Education, to be appointed by the Central Government.

• One person to represent the Indian Board for Wild Life, to be appointed by the Central Government.

• Three persons who, in the opinion of the Central Government, are or have been actively engaged in animal welfare work and are well-known humanitarians, to be nominated by the Central Government.

(c) One person to represent such association of veterinary practitioners as in the opinion of the Central Government ought to be represented on the Board, to be elected by that association in the prescribed manner.

(d) Two persons to represent practitioners of modern and indigenous systems of medicine, to be nominated by the Central Government.

(e) One person to represent each of such two municipal corporations as in the opinion of the Central Government ought to be represented on the Board, to be elected by each of the said corporations in the prescribed manner.

(f) One person to represent each of such three organisations actively interested in animal welfare as in the opinion of the Central Government ought to be represented on the Board, to be chosen by each of the said organisations in the prescribed manner.

(g) One person to represent each of such three societies dealing with prevention of cruelty to animal as in the opinion of the Central Government ought to be represented on the Board, to be chosen, in the prescribed manner.

(h) Three persons to be nominated by the Central Government.

(i) Six Members of Parliament, four to be elected by the House of the People (Lok Sabha) and two by the Council of States (Rajya Sabha).

2.   Any of the persons referred to in clause 9(a) or clause (b) or clause (ba) or clause (bb) of sub-section (1) may depute any other person to attend any of the meetings of the Board.

3.   The Central Government shall nominate one of the members of the Board to be its Chairman and another member of the Board to be its Vice-Chairman.

RECONSTITUTION OF THE BOARD

1.   In order that the Chairman and other members of the Board hold office till the same date and that their terms of office come to an end on the same date, the Central Government may, by notification in the Official Gazette, reconstitute, as soon as may be after the Prevention of Cruelty to Animals (Amendment) Act, 1982 comes into force, the Board.

2.   The Board as reconstituted under sub-section (1) shall be reconstituted from time to time on the expiration of every third year, from the date of its reconstitution under sub-section (1).

3.   There shall be included amongst the members of the Board reconstituted under sub section (1), all persons who immediately before the date on which such reconstitution is to take effect, are Members of the Board but such persons shall hold office only for

the unexpired portion of the term for which they would have held office if such reconstitution had not been made and the vacancies arising as a result of their ceasing to be Members of the Board shall be filled up as casual vacancies for the remaining period of the term of the Board as so reconstituted.

Provided that nothing in this sub-section shall apply in relation to any person who ceases to be member of the Board by virtue of the amendment made in sub-section (1) of section 5 by sub-clause (ii) of clause (a) of section 5 of the Prevention of Cruelty to Animals (Amendment) Act, 1982.

TERM OF OFFICE AND CONDITIONS OF SERVICE OF MEMBERS OF THE BOARD

1. The term for which the Board may be reconstituted under section 5A shall be three years from the date of the reconstitution and the Chairman and other Members of the Board as so reconstituted shall hold office till the expiry of the term for which the Board has been so reconstituted.

2. Notwithstanding anything contained in sub-section (1),

(a) The term of office of an ex-officio Member shall continue so long as he holds the office by virtue of which he is such a Member;

(b) The term of office of a Member elected or chosen under clause (c), clause (e), clause (g), clause (h) or clause (i) of section 5 to represent anybody of persons shall come to an end as soon as he ceases to be a Member of the body which elected him or in respect of which he was chosen;

(c) The term of office of a Member appointed, nominated, elected or chosen to fill a casual vacancy shall continue for the remainder of the term of office of the Member in whose place he is appointed, nominated, elected or chosen;

(d) The Central Government may, at any time, remove for reasons to be recorded in writing a member from office after giving him a reasonable opportunity of showing cause against the proposed removal and any vacancy caused by such removal shall be treated as casual vacancy for the purpose of clause (c).

3.   The members of the Board shall receive such allowance, if any, as the Board may, subject to the previous approval of the Central Government, provided by regulations made in this behalf,

4.   No act done or proceeding taken by the Board shall be questioned on the ground merely of the existence of any vacancy in, or defect in the constitution of the Board and in particular, and without prejudice to the generality of the foregoing, during the period intervening between the expiry of the term for which the Board has been reconstituted under section 5A and its further reconstitution under that section, the ex-officio members of the Board shall discharge all the powers and function of the Board.

SECRETARY AND OTHER EMPLOYEES OF THE BOARD

1.   The Central Government shall appoint the Secretary of the Board.

2.   Subject to such rules as may be made by the Central Government in this behalf, the Board may appoint such number of other officers and employees as may be necessary for the exercise of its powers and the discharge of its functions and may determine the terms and conditions of service of such officers and other employees by regulations made by it with the previous approval of the Central Government.

8.3 FUNCTIONS OF THE BOARD

The functions of the Board shall be Board are,

1.   To keep the law in force in, India for the prevention of cruelty to animals under constant study and advice the Government on the amendments to be undertaken in any such law from time to time.

2.   To advise the Central Government on the making of rules under this Act with a view to preventing unnecessary pain or suffering to animals generally, and more particularly when they are being transported from one place to another or when they are used as

performing animals or when they are kept in captivity or confinement.

3. To advise the Government or any local authority or other person on improvements in the design of vehicles so as to lessen the burden on draught animals.

4. To take all such steps as the Board may think fit for amelioration of animals by encouraging or providing for, the construction of sheds, water-troughs and the like and by providing for veterinary assistance to animals.

5. To advise the Government or any local authority or other person in the design of slaughter-houses or the maintenance of slaughter houses or in connection with slaughter of animals so that unnecessary pain or suffering, whether physical or mental, is eliminated in the pre-slaughter stages as far as possible, and animals are killed; wherever necessary, in as humane a manner as possible.

6. To take all such steps as the Board may think fit to ensure that unwanted animals are destroyed by local authorities, whenever it is necessary to do so, either instantaneously or after being rendered insensible to pain or suffering.

7. To encourage by the grant of financial assistance or otherwise, the formation or establishment of pinjrapoles, rescue homes, animal shelters, sanctuaries and the like where animals and birds may find a shelter when they have become old and useless or when they need protection.

8. to co-operate with, and co-ordinate the work of, associations or bodies established for the purpose of preventing unnecessary pain or suffering to animals or for the protection of animals and birds.

9. To give financial and other assistance to animal welfare organisations functioning in any local area or to encourage the formation of animal welfare organisations in any local area this shall work under the general supervision and guidance of the Board.

10. To advise the Government on matters relating to the medical care and attention which may be provided in animal hospital, and to give financial and other assistance to animal hospitals whenever the Board thinks it necessary to do so.

11. to impart education in relation to the humane treatment of animals and to encourage the formation of public opinion against the infliction of unnecessary pain or suffering to animals and for the promotion of animal welfare by means of lectures, books, posters, cinematographic exhibitions and the like.

12. To advise the Government on any matter connected with animal welfare or the prevention of infliction of unnecessary pain or suffering on animals.

8.4 CRUELTY TO ANIMALS

Treating animals cruelly

1. If any person,

(a) Beats, kicks, over-rides, over-drives, over-loads, tortures or otherwise treats any animal so as to subject it to unnecessary pain or suffering or causes, or being the owner permits, any animal to be so treated; or

(b) Employs in any work or labour or for any purpose any animal which, by reason of its age or any disease infirmity; wound, sore or other cause, is unfit to be so employed or, being the owner, permits any such unfit animal to be employed; or

(c) Wilfully and unreasonably administers any injurious drug or injurious substance to any animal or wilfully and unreasonably causes or attempts to cause any such drug or substance to be taken by any animal; or

(d) Conveys or carries, whether in or upon any vehicle or not, any animal in such a manner or position as to subject it to unnecessary pain or suffering; or

(e) Keeps or confines any animal in any -cage or other receptacle which does not measure sufficiently in height, length and breadth to permit the animal a reasonable opportunity for movement; or

(f) Keeps for an unreasonable time any animal chained or tethered upon an unreasonably short or unreasonably heavy chain or cord; or

(g) Being the owner, neglects to exercise or cause to be exercised reasonably any dog habitually chained up or kept in close confinement; or

(h) Being the owner of any animal fails to provide such animal with sufficient food, drink or shelter; or

(i) Without reasonable cause, abandons any animal in circumstances which tender it likely that it will suffer pain by reason of starvation thirst; or

(j) Wilfully permits any animal, of which he is the owner, to go at large in any street, while the animal is affected with contagious or infectious disease or, without reasonable excuse permits any diseased or disabled animal, of which he is the owner, to die in any street; or

(k) Offers for sale or without reasonable cause, has in his possession any animal which is suffering pain by reason of mutilation, starvation, thirst, overcrowding or other ill-treatment; or

(l) Mutilates any animal or kills any animal (including stray dogs) by using the method of strychnine injections, in the heart or in any other unnecessarily cruel manner or,

(m) Solely with a view to providing entertainment

• Confines or causes to be confined any animal including tying of an animal as a bait in a tiger or other sanctuary so as to make it an object or prey for any other animal; or

(n) Organises, keeps uses or acts in the management or, any place for animal fighting or for the purpose of baiting any animal or permits or offers any place to be so used or receives money for the admission of any other person to any place kept or used for any such purposes; or

(o) Promotes or takes part in any shooting match or competition wherein animals are released from captivity for the purpose of such shooting: he shall be punishable in the case of a first offence, with fine which shall not be less than ten rupees but which may extend to fifty rupees and in the case of a second or subsequent offence committed within three years of the previous offence, with fine which shall not be less than twenty-five rupees but which may extend, to one hundred rupees or with imprisonment for a term which may extend, to three months, or with both.

2.   For the purposes of section (1) an owner shall be deemed to have committed an offence if he has failed to exercise reasonable care and supervision with a view to the prevention of such offence;

Provided that where an owner is convicted permitting cruelty by reason only of having failed to exercise such care and supervision, he shall not be liable to imprisonment without the option of a fine.

3.   Nothing in this section shall apply to-

(a) The dehorning of cattle, or the castration or branding or nose roping of any animal in the prescribed manner, or

(b) The destruction of stray dogs in lethal chambers by such other methods as may be prescribed or

(c) The extermination or destruction of any animal under the authority of any law for the time being in force; or

(d) Any matter dealt with in Chapter IV; or

(e) The commission or omission of any act in the course of the destruction or the preparation for destruction of any animal as food for mankind unless such destruction or preparation was accompanied by the infliction of unnecessary pain or suffering.

8.5 EXPERIMENTATION OF ANIMALS

This Act shall control performance of experiments, including experiments involving operations on animals for the purpose of advancement by new discovery of physiological knowledge or of knowledge which will be useful for saving or, for prolonging life or alleviating suffering or for combating any disease, whether of human beings, animals or plants.

Committee for control and supervision of experiments on animals

1. If at any time, on the advice of the Board, the Central Government is of opinion that it is necessary so to do for the purpose of controlling "and supervising experiments on animals it may be notification in the Official Gazette.

Constitute a Committee consisting of such number of officials and non-officials, as it may think fit to appoint thereto.

2. The Central Government shall nominate one of the Members of the Committee to be its Chairman.

3. The Committee shall have power to regulate its own Procedure in relation to the performance of its duties.

4. The funds of the Committee shall consist of grants made to it from time to time by the Government and of contributions, donations, subscriptions, bequests, gifts and the like made to it by any person..

Sub-Committee

1. The Committee may constitute as many sub-committees as it thinks fit for exercising any power or discharging any duty of the Committee or for inquiring into or reporting and advising on any matter which the Committee may refer.

2. A sub-committee shall consist exclusively of the Members of the Committee.

Staff of the Committee

Subject to the control of the Central Government, the Committee may appoint such number of officers and other employees as may be necessary to enable it to exercise ills powers and perform its duties and may determine the remuneration and other terms and conditions of service of such officers and other employees.

Duties of the Committee and power of the Committee to make rules relating to

Experiments on animals

1.   It shall be the duty of the Committee to take all such measures as may be necessary to ensure that animals are not subjected to unnecessary pain or suffering before, during or after the performance of experiments on them, and for the purpose it may, by notification in the Gazette of India and subject to the condition of previous publication, make such rules as it may think fit in animals relation to the conduct of such experiments.

2.   In particular, and without prejudice to the generality to the foregoing power, such rules may provide for the following matters namely-

    (a) The registration of persons or institutions carrying on experiments on animals.

    (b) The reports and other information which shall be forwarded to the Committee by persons and institutions carrying on experiments or, animals.

3.   In particular, and without prejudice to the generality of the foregoing power, rules made by the Committee shall be designed to secure the following objects, namely.

    (a) In cases where experiments are performed in any institution, the responsibility therefore is placed on the person in charge of the institution and that, in cases where experiments are performed outside an institution by individuals, the individuals, are performed outside an institution by individuals, the individuals, are qualified in that behalf and the experiments are performed on their full responsibility.

(b) Experiments are performed with due care and humanity and that as far as possible experiments involving operations are performed under the influence of some anaesthetic of sufficient power to prevent the animals feeling pain.

(c) Animals which, in the course of experiments under the influence of anaesthetics, are so injured that their recovery would involve serious suffering, are ordinarily destroyed while still insensible.

(d) Experiments on animals are avoided wherever it is possible to do so; as for example; in medical schools, hospitals, colleges and the like, if other teaching devices such as books, models, films and the. like, may equally suffice.

(e) Experiments on larger animals are avoided when it is possible to achieve the same results by experiments upon small laboratory animals like guinea-'pigs, rabbits, frogs and rats.

(f) As far as possible, experiments are not performed merely for the purpose of acquiring manual skill.

(g) Animals intended for the performance of experiments are properly looked after both before and after experiments.

(h) Suitable records are maintained with respect to experiments performed on animals.

4.   In making any rules under this section, the Committee shall be guided by such directions as the Central Government (consistently with the objects for which the Committee is set up) may give to it, and the Central Government is hereby authorised to give such direction.

5.   All rules made by the Committee shall be binding on all individuals performing experiments outside institutions and one person in charge of institutions in which experiments are performed.

Power of entry and inspection

For the purpose of ensuring that the rules made by it are being complied and with the Committee may authorise any of its officers or any other person in writing to inspect any institution or place where experiments are being carried on and report to it as a result of such inspection, and any officer or person so authorised may-

(a) Enter at any time considered reasonable by him and inspect any institution or place in which experiments on animals are being carried on; and

(b) Require any person to produce any record kept by him with respect to experiments on animals.

Power to prohibit experiments on animals

If the Committee is satisfied, on the report of any officer or other person made to it as a result of any inspection under section 18 or otherwise that the rules made by it under section 17 are not being animals the Committee may, after giving an opportunity to the person or institution carrying on experiments on animals; the Committee may, after giving an opportunity to the person or institution of being heard in the matter, by order, prohibit the person or institution from carrying on any such experiments either for a specified period or indefinitely, or may allow the person or institution to carry on such experiments subject to such special conditions as the Committee may think fit to impose.

Penalties

If any person-

(a) Contravenes any order made by the Committee under section 19; or

(b) Commits a breach of any condition imposed by the Committee under that section: he shall be punishable with fine which may extend to two hundred rupees, and, when the contravention or breach of condition has taken place in any institution the person in charge of the institution shall be deemed to be guilty of the offence and shall be punishable accordingly.

PART B

AP SHOPS AND ESTABLISHMENTS ACT 1988

AND RULE 1990

8.6 INTRODUCTION

1.   This Act may be called Andhra Pradesh Shops and Establishments Act, 1988.

2.   It extends to the whole of the State of Andhra Pradesh.

3.   It shall come into force on such date as the Government may, by notification, appoint.

4.   It shall apply-

a)   In the first instance to all areas in which the Andhra Pradesh Shops and Establishments Act, 1966 was in force immediately before the commencement of this Act;

b)   To such other areas in the State on such date as the Government may, by notification, specify.

DEFINITIONS

1.   *Apprentice:* Means a person who is employed whether on payment of wages or not, for the purpose of being trained in any trade, craft or employment in any establishment;

2.   *Chief Inspector:* Means the Chief Inspector appointed under Section 57;

3.   *Child means:* A person who has not completed fourteen years of age;

4.   *Close:* Means not open for the service of any customer, or for any trade or business or for any other purpose connected with the establishment except loading, unloading and annual stock taking;

5.   *Commercial Establishment:* Means an establishment which carries on any trade, business, profession or any work in connection

with or incidental or ancilliary to any such trade, business or profession or which is a clerical department of a factory or an industrial undertaking or which is a commercial or trading or banking or insurance establishment and includes an establishment under the management and control of a co operative society, an establishment of a factory or an industrial undertaking which falls outside the scope of the Factories Act, 1948, (Central Act 63 of 1948), and such other establishment as the Government may, by notification declare to be a commercial establishment for the purposes of this Act but does not include a shop;

6.   *Day:* Means the period of twenty four hours beginning at mid night:

Provided that, in the case of an employee, whose hours of work extend beyond mid night, day means the period of twenty four hours beginning from the time when such employment commences.

7.   *Dependant:* Means in relation to a deceased employee, his nominee or in the absence of such nominee, the heir or legal representative;

8.   *Employee:* Means a person wholly or principally employed in, and in connection with, any establishment and includes an apprentice and any clerical or other staff of a factory or industrial establishment who fall outside the scope of the Factories Act, 1948; (Central Act, 63 of 1948) but does not include the husband, wife, son, daughter, father, mother, brother or sister of an employer or his partner, who is living with and depending upon such employer or partner and is not in receipt of any wages;

9.   *Employer:* Means a person having charge of or owning or having ultimate control over the affairs of an establishment and includes the Manager, agent or other person acting in the general management or control of an establishment;

10.   *Establishment:* Means a shop, restaurant, eating house, residential hotel, lodging house, theatre or any place of public amusement or entertainment and includes a commercial establishment and such other establishment as the Government may, by notification, declare to be an establishment for the purpose of this Act;

11. **Factory:** Means a factory within the meaning of the Factories Act, 1948, (Central Act 63 of 1948);

12. **Inspector:** Means an Inspector appointed under Section 50;

13. **Notification:** Means a notification published in the Andhra Pradesh Gazette and the word notified , shall be construed accordingly;

14. **Opened:** Means opened for the service of any customer or for any trade or business connected with the establishment;

15. **Periods of work:** Means the time during which an employee is at the disposal of the employer;

16. **Prescribed:** Means prescribed by rules made by the Government under this Act;

17. **Register of establishment:** Means a register maintained for the registration of establishment under this Act;

18. **Registration certificate:** Means a certificate issued under this Act;

19. **Service:** Compensation means the service compensation payable under Section 40;

20. **Shop:** Means any premises where any trade or business is carried on or where services are rendered to customers and includes a shop run by a Co operative Society, an office, a store room, godown, warehouse or work place, whether in the same premises or otherwise, used in connection with such trade or business and such other establishments as the Government may, by notification, declare to be a shop for the purposes of this Act, but does not include a commercial establishment;

21. **Wages:** Means every remuneration, whether by way of salary, allowance, or otherwise expressed in terms of money or capable of being so expressed which would, if the terms of employment, express or implied were fulfilled, be payable to an employee in respect of his employment or of work done in such employment, and includes

a)   Any remuneration payable under any settlement, between the parties or order of a tribunal or court;

b)   Any remuneration to which the employee is entitled in respect of overtime work or holidays or any leave period;

c)   Any additional remuneration payable under the terms of employment, whether called a bonus or by any other name;

d)   Any sum which by reason of the termination of employment of the employee is payable under any law, contract or instrument which provides for the payment of such sum, whether with or without deductions, but does not provide for the time within which the payment is to be made;

e)   Any sum to which the employee is entitled under any scheme framed under any law for the time being in force; but does not include

i.   Any bonus, whether under a scheme of profit sharing or otherwise, which does not form part of the remuneration payable under the terms of employment or which is not payable under any award or settlement between the parties or order of court

ii.   The value of any house accommodation, or of the supply of light, water, medical attendance or other amenity or of any service excluded from the computation of wages by a general or special order of the Government;

iii.   Any contribution paid by the employer to any person or provident fund, and the interest which may have accrued thereon;

iv.   Any travelling allowance or the value of any travelling concession;

v.   Any sum paid to the employee to defray special expenses entailed on him by the nature of his employment

vi.   Any service compensation payable on the termination of employment in cases other than those specified in sub clause

vii.   The subscription paid by the employee to life insurance and contribution paid by the employer to the life insurance of the employee under the provisions of this Act and the bonus which may have accrued thereon; or

viii.   House rent allowance payable by the employer;

22. **Week:** Means a period of seven days beginning at mid night on Saturday;

23. **Young Person:** Means a person who is not a child and has not completed eighteen years of age.

8.7 REGISTRATION OF ESTABLISHMENTS

1. Every employer of an establishment shall,

    a)   In the case of an establishment existing on the date of commencement of this Act, within thirty days from that date; and

    b)   In the case of a new establishment, within thirty days from the date on which the establishment commences its work, send to the Inspector concerned a statement containing such particulars, together with such fees, as may be prescribed.

2. On receipt of such statement, the Inspector shall register the establishment in the register of establishments in such manner as may be prescribed and shall issue in the prescribed form a registration certificate to the employer who shall display it at a prominent place of the establishment.

3. Every registration certificate issued under sub section (2), shall be valid with effect from the date on which it is issued up to the 31st day of December following.

4. Every employer shall give intimation to the Inspector, in the prescribed form, any change in any of the particulars in the statement made under sub section (1) within fifteen days after the change has taken place. The Inspector shall, on receipt of such intimation and the fees prescribed therefor make the change in the register of establishments in accordance with such intimation and shall amend the registration certificate or issue a fresh registration certificate, if necessary.

5. The employer shall, within fifteen days of the closure of the establishment, give intimation thereof in writing to the Inspector,

who shall, on receipt of such intimation, remove the name of the establishment from the register of establishments and cancel the registration certificate:

Provided that, where the Inspector is satisfied otherwise than on receipt of such intimation, that the establishment has been closed, he shall remove the name of such establishment from the register and cancel the registration certificate.

Renewal of Registration Certificates

1.   The Inspector may, on an application made by the employer accompanied by the fees prescribed therefor, renew the registration certificate for a period of one year or for such number of years as may be prescribed, commencing from the date of its expiry.

2.   Every application for the renewal of the registration certificate shall be made in such form and in such manner as may be prescribed so as to reach the Inspector not later than thirty days before the date of its expiry:

    Provided that, an application for the renewal of a registration certificate received not later than thirty days after its expiry may be entertained by the Inspector on the applicant paying such penalty as may be prescribed, by the Government from time to time.

3.   An applicant for the renewal of a registration certificate under sub section (2) shall, until communication of orders on his application, be entitled to act as if the registration certificate had been renewed.

Revocation or suspension of the Registration Certificate

    If the Inspector is satisfied, either on a reference made to him in this behalf or otherwise, that

a)   The Registration Certificate granted under Section 3 or renewed under Section 4 has been obtained by misrepresentation, fraud or suppression of any material fact; or

b)   The employer has wilfully contravened any of the provisions of this Act or the Rules made thereunder. The Inspector may without prejudice to any other penalty to which the employer may be liable under this Act, revoke or suspend the Registration Certificate, after giving the employer an opportunity of showing cause.

Appeal against revocation or suspension of the Registration certificate

a) Any person aggrieved by an order made under Section 5 may, within thirty days from the date on which the order is communicated to him, prefer an appeal to such authority as may be prescribed:

Provided that the appellate authority may entertain the appeal after the expiry of the said period of thirty days if he is satisfied that the appellant was prevented by sufficient cause from the filing the appeal in time.

b) On receipt of an appeal under sub section (1), the appellate authority shall, after giving the appellant an opportunity of being heard, dispose of the appeal within two months.

8.8 SHOP

Opening and closing hours of shops

a) No shop shall on any day be opened earlier or closed later than such hour as may, after previous publication, be fixed by the Government by a general or special order in that behalf:

Provided that, any customer who was being served or was waiting to be served in any shop at the hour fixed for its closing may be served during the quarter of an hour immediately following such hour.

b) The Government may, for the purposes of this section, fix different hours for different classes of shops or for different areas or for different time of the year.

Selling outside prohibited before opening and after closing hours of shops

No person shall carry on, in or adjacent to, a street or public place, the sale of any goods, before the opening and after the closing hours fixed under Section 7 for the shops dealing in any kind of goods in the locality in which such street or public place is situated:

Provided that, nothing in this section shall apply to the sale of

a) Newspapers.

b) Flowers.

c) Pan

d) Vegetables and fruits; and

e) Such other goods as the Government may, by notification, specify from time to time.

Daily and weekly hours of work in shops

1. Subject to other provisions of this Act, no employee in any shop shall be required or allowed to work therein for more than eight hours in any day and forty eight hours in any week.

2. Any employee may be required or allowed to work in a shop for any period in excess of the limit fixed under sub section (1), on payment of overtime wages, subject to a maximum period of six hours in a week.

3. For the purpose of stock taking and preparation of accounts, an employer may, with the previous intimation to the Inspector, require or allow any employee to work in a shop for not more than any six days in a year in excess of the period fixed in sub section (1), on payment of overtime wages; so however, that the excess period shall not in aggregate exceed twenty four hours

Interval for rest

No employee in any shop shall be required or allowed to work therein for more than five hours in any day unless he has had an interval for rest of at least one hour:

Provided that, an employee who was serving a customer at the commencement of the interval may be required to serve him during the quarter of an hour immediately following such commencement.

Spread over periods of work

The periods of work of an employee in a shop shall be so arranged that along with his intervals for rest, they shall not spread over for more than twelve hours in any day

Provided that, where an employee works on any day for the purpose of stock taking and preparation of accounts, the spread over shall not exceed fourteen hours in any such day on payment of overtime wages.

Closing of shops and grant of holidays

1. Every shop, whether with or without employees, shall remain closed on every Sunday which shall be a holiday for every employee in the shop:

   Provided that the Chief Inspector may, by notification, specify in respect of any shop or class of shops or in respect of shops or class of shops in any area any day in the week instead of Sunday on which day such shop or class of shops shall remain closed. .

   (a) The Chief Inspector may, by notification, require in respect of any specified class of shops that they shall in addition to the weekly holiday mentioned in sub section (1), be closed for one half day in a week, as may be fixed by the Government;

   (b) Every employee in any shop to which a notification under Clause (a) applies, shall be allowed in each week an additional holiday of one half day fixed for the closing of the shop under Clause (a).

2. The Chief Inspector may, for the purposes of sub section (2), fix different hours for different classes of shops or for different areas or for different times of the year.

3. The weekly day on which a shop is closed in pursuance of a requirement under sub section (2) shall be specified by the employer in a notice prominently exhibited in a conspicuous place in the shop.

4. It shall not be lawful for the employer to call an employee at or for the employee to go to his shop or any place for any work in connection with the business of his shop on any day or part of the day on which it has remained closed.

5. No deduction shall be made from the wages of any employee in a shop on account of any day or part of a day on which it has remained closed; and if such employee is employed on the basis that he would not ordinarily receive wages for such day or part of a day he shall nonetheless be paid for such day or part of a day the wages he would have drawn had the shop not remained closed, or had the holiday not been allowed, on that day or part of a day.

Closing of shops in public interest during special occasions

In addition to the holidays mentioned in Section 12, the Chief Inspector may, by notification, and with the previous approval of the Government, require in respect of any specified class of shops that they shall be closed on any specified day or days in the public interest.

8.9 ESTABLISHMENTS OTHER THAN SHOPS

Application of this Chapter to establishments other than shops:

The provisions of this Chapter shall apply only to establishments other than shops.

Opening and closing hours

1. No establishment shall on any day be opened earlier, or closed later, than such hour as may, after previous publication, be fixed by the Government by general or special order in that behalf:

    Provided that, in the case of a restaurant or eating house, any customer who was being served or was waiting to be served therein at the hour fixed for its closing may be served during the quarter of an hour immediately following such hour.

2. The Government may, for the purpose of this section, fix different hours for different classes of establishments or for different areas or for different times of the year.

Daily and weekly hours of work

1. Subject to the provisions of this Act, no employee in any establishment shall be required or allowed to work therein for more than eight hours in any day and forty eight hours in any week.

2. Any employee may required or allowed to work in an establishment for any period in excess of the limit fixed under sub section (1), on payment of overtime wages, subject to a maximum period of six hours in any week.

3. For the purposes of stock taking and preparation of accounts, an employer may, with the previous intimation to the Inspector, require or allow any employee to work in an establishment for not more than any six days in a year in excess of the period fixed in sub section (1) on payment of overtime wages; so however, that the excess period shall not, in the aggregate, exceed twenty four hours.

Interval for rest

No employee in any establishment shall be required or allowed to work in such establishment for more than five hours in any day unless he has had an interval for rest of at least one hour.

Provided that the Chief Inspector may, in the case of an establishment whose daily hours of work are less than eight hours, reduce interval for rest to half an hour on an application made by the employer, with the consent of the employees.

Spread over of periods of work

The periods of work of an employee in an establishment shall be so arranged that, along with his interval for rest, they shall not spread over for more than twelve hours on any day:

Provided that, where an employee works on any day for the purpose of stock taking and preparation of accounts the spread over shall not exceed fourteen hours on any such day on payment of over time wage.

Holidays

1. Every employee in any establishment shall be allowed in each week a holiday of one whole day:

Provided that, nothing in this sub section shall apply to any employee whose total period of employment in the week, including any days spent on authorised leave is less than six days.

2.   The Government may, by notification, require in respect of any specified class of establishments that every employee therein shall be allowed in each week an additional holiday of one half day commencing at such hour in the afternoon as may be fixed by the Government.

3.   The Government may, for the purposes of sub section (2) fix different hours for different classes of establishments or for different areas or for different times of the year.

4.   No deduction shall be made from the wages of any employee in an establishment on account of any day or part of a day on which a holiday has been allowed in accordance with this section and if such employee is employed on the basis that he would not ordinarily receive wages for such day or part of a day, he shall nonetheless be paid for such day or part of a day the wages he would have drawn, had the holiday not been allowed on that day or part of a day.

5.   It shall not be lawful for the employer to call an employee at or for the employee to go to, his establishment or any other place for any work in connection with the business of his establishment on any day or part of a day on which a holiday has been allowed in accordance with this section.

8.10 EMPLOYMENT OF WOMEN, CHILDREN AND YOUNG PERSONS

1.   Children not to work in establishment: No child shall be required or allowed to work in any establishment.

2.   Special provision for young person: No young person shall be required or allowed to work in establishment before 6 a.m. and after 7 p.m.

3.   Daily and weekly hours of work for young person: Notwithstanding anything in this Act, no young person shall be required or allowed to work in any establishment for more than 7 hours in any day and forty two hours in any week nor shall such person be allowed to work overtime.

4. Special provision for women: No Woman employee shall be required or allowed to work in any establishment before 6:00 a.m. and after 8:30 p.m.

5. Maternity leave: The periods of absence from duty in respect of which a woman employee is entitled to maternity benefit under Section 25, shall be treated as authorised absence from duty, and the woman employee shall be entitled to maternity benefit, but not to any wages for any of those periods.

6. Maternity Benefit: Every woman who has been for a period of not less than six months preceding the date of her delivery in continuous employment of the same employer whether in the same or different shops or commercial establishments, shall be entitled to receive from her employer for the period of

a) Six weeks immediately preceding the day of delivery; and

b) Six weeks following the day of delivery; such maternity benefit and in such manner as may be prescribed:

Provided that, no woman employee shall be entitled to receive such benefit for any day during any of the aforesaid periods, on which she attends work and receive wages therefor

8.11 HEALTH AND SAFETY

1. Cleanliness: The premises of every establishment shall be kept clean and free from effluvia arising from any drain or privy or other nuisance and shall be cleaned at such times and by such methods as may be prescribed.

2. Ventilation: The premises of every establishment shall be ventilated as provided for in the laws relating to the municipalities, Gram Panchayats or other local authorities for the time being in force.

3. Precautions for the safety of employees in establishments:

a) In every establishment other than such establishment or class of establishments as the Governments may, by notification, specify, such precautions against fire shall be taken as may be prescribed.

b)   If power driven machinery is used, or any process which, in the opinion of the Government, is likely to expose any employee to a serious risk of bodily injury is carried on in any establishment, such precautions including the keeping of first aid box shall be taken by the employer for the safety of the employees therein, as may be prescribed.

4.   Maximum permissible load

a)   No employee in any establishment shall be required or allowed to engage in the manual transport of a load therein which by reason of its weight is likely to jeopardise his health or safety.

b)   The Government may, for the purposes of this section prescribe different maximum limits of weight, for different classes of employees in any establishment.

8.12 LEAVE AND HOLIDAYS WITH WAGES AND INSURANCE SCHEME FOR EMPLOYEES

Leaves

1.   Every employee who has served for a period of two hundred and forty days or more during a continuous period of twelve months in any establishment shall be entitled during the subsequent period of twelve months, to leave with wages for period of fifteen days, provided that such leave with wages may be accumulated up to a maximum period of sixty days.

2.   An employee may apply in writing to the employer, not less than seven full working days before the date of availing himself of his leave, to allow all the leave or any portion thereof, to which he is entitled under sub section (1).

3.   An employee, who has been allowed leave for not less than five days under sub section (2) shall, before his leave begins, be paid the wages due for the period of the leave allowed if he makes a request therefor.

4.   Every employee who has served for a period of not less than two hundred and forty days during a continuous period of twelve months

in any establishment shall be entitled for encashment of eight days of leave with wages that has accrued to him under sub section (1) during the subsequent period of twelve months. The employer shall pay to the employee the wages for the leave so encashed by the employee within a week of receipt of the application for such encashment from the employee.

5. Every employee in any establishment shall also be entitled during his first twelve months of continuous service and during every subsequent twelve months of service,

a) To leave with wages for a period not exceeding twelve days on the ground of any sickness or accident and

b) To casual leave with wages for a period not exceeding twelve days on any reasonable ground.

6. Every employee in an establishment after he has put in not less than two years of service under the same employer, shall also be entitled for special casual leave not exceeding six days only once during his entire service, if he has undergone vasectomy or tubectomy operation, subject to the production of a certificate therefor from an authorised medical practitioner under whom he has undergone the operation.

7. If any employee entitled to any leave under sub section (1) is discharged by his employer before he has been allowed such leave, or if the leave applied for by such employee has been refused and if he quits his employment before he has been allowed the leave, the employer shall pay him the amount, payable under this Act, in respect of the period of leave.

8. If an employee is lawfully discharged by his employer when he is sick or suffering from the result of an accident the employer shall pay him the amount payable under this Act in respect of the period of leave to which he was entitled at the time of his discharge in addition to the amount, if any, payable to him under sub section (3).

9. An employee in a hostel attached to a school or college or in an establishment maintained in connection with the boarding and lodging

of pupils and resident masters, shall be allowed the privileges referred to in sub sections (1) to (8), reduced however proportionately to the period for which he was employed continuously in the previous year or to the period for which he will be employed continuously in the current year, as the case may be; and all references to the periods of leave in sub sections (1) and (5) shall be construed accordingly, fractions of less than half a day being disregarded.

Other holidays

1. Every employee in any establishment shall also be entitled to nine holidays in a year with wages on the days to be specified by notification from time to time, by the Government which shall include the 26th January (Republic day), 1st May, (May Day), 15th August (Independence Day) 2nd October (Gandhi Jayanthi), and 1st November (Andhra Pradesh Formation Day) and on every such holiday, all the establishments, either with or without employees, shall remain closed.

2. Notwithstanding anything contained in sub section (1) the Chief Inspector may, having due regard to any emergency or special circumstances prevailing in the State or any part thereof, notify any other day or days as holidays with wages to employees or class of employees as he may deem fit. The holidays so notified shall be deemed to be additional holidays.

3. Nothing in sub section (1) shall apply in respect of any establishment where the number of holidays with wages allowed by the employer is more than the holidays notified by the Government under that sub section.

Pay during leave and holidays

Every employee shall, for the period of the leave allowed under sub sections (1) (5) of Section 30 or the holidays allowed under Section 31, be paid at a rate equivalent to the daily average of his wages for the days on which he actually worked during the preceding month exclusive of any earning in respect of overtime.

Power to increase the period of leave allowable under Section 30

Notwithstanding anything in Section 30, the Government may, by notification, increase the total number of days of leave allowable under sub section (1) of that section and the maximum number of days upto which such leave may be accumulated in respect of any establishment or class of establishments.

Compulsory enrolment of employees to Insurance cum savings scheme

1. Every employee who has served in an establishment for a period of not less than one year shall subscribe to the insurance scheme or Insurance cum Savings scheme as may be notified by the Government to be applicable to the establishment in which the employee is working, at the rates, stipulated by the Government in the notification either in lumpsum every year or in monthly instalments as may be prescribed by the Government in the notification. For this purpose the employer shall make the payment to the authority notified by the Government on behalf of the employee on or before the stipulated date and recover the same from the wages payable to the employee.

2. In addition to the subscription of the employee mentioned in sub section (1), every employer of the establishment to which the scheme of insurance or Insurance cum Savings is made applicable by the Government, shall also pay such percentage of annual wages of employee as may be notified by the Government, from time to time, to the authority notified for the purpose as employer s contribution on or before the specified date every year.

8.13 WAGES

1. Responsibility for payment of wages: Every employer shall be responsible for the payment by him to employees of all wages and sums, required to be paid under this Act.

2. Fixation of wage period:

   a) Every employer shall fix periods (hereinafter referred to as wage periods) in respect of which such wages shall be payable.

b)   No wage period shall exceed one month.

3.   Wages for overtime work: Where any employee in any establishment is required to work over time he shall be entitled, in respect of such overtime work, to wages at twice the ordinary rate of wages.

4.   Time of payment of wages:

a)   The wages of every employee shall be paid before the expiry of the fifth day after the last day of the wage period in respect of which the wages are payable.

b)   Where the service of any employee is terminated by or on behalf of the employer the wages earned by such employee shall be paid before the expiration of the second working day from the day on which his employment is terminated.

c)   The Government may, by general or special order and for reasons stated therein exempt an employer from the operation of this section in respect of the wages of any employee or class of employees to such extent and subject to such conditions as may be specified in the order.

d)   All payments of wages shall be made on a working day.

5.   Wages to be paid in current coin or currency notes: All wages shall be paid in current coin or currency notes or in both.

8.14 APPOINTMENT, POWERS AND DUTIES OF THE CHIEF INSPECTOR AND INSPECTORS

1.   Appointment of Chief Inspector and Inspectors: The Government may, by notification, appoint a Chief Inspector and such number of Inspectors as may be necessary for the purposes of this Act and fix the local limits of their jurisdiction.

2.   Powers and duties of Chief Inspector: The Chief Inspector may exercise and perform in addition to the powers and duties conferred and imposed on him by or under this Act, all the powers and duties of an Inspector under this Act.

3.   Powers and duties of Inspectors: An Inspector may, within the local limits for which he is appointed,

a)   Enter at all reasonable hours with the assistance of such persons in the service of the Government or any local authority as he thinks fit, any place which is or which he has reason to believe is used as an establishment;

b)   Make such inspection of the premises and of any registers or other records and take on the spot or otherwise evidence of such persons, as he may deem necessary in the manner prescribed;

c)   Exercise such other powers as may be necessary for carrying out of the purposes of this Act.

4.   Chief Inspector and Inspectors to be public servants: The Chief Inspector and every Inspector shall be deemed to be public servants within the meaning of Section 21 of the Indian Penal Code.

PENALTIES FOR OFFENCES

S.no	OFFENCES	PENALTIES
1.	Anyone who makes false entry or omits any entry.	3 months imprisonment and or fine from Rs 50/- to Rs 250/-
2.	Anyone who obstructs an inspector or prevents employee appearing before an inspector.	Fine from Rs 50/- to Rs 250/
3.	Anyone who fails to keep records or display notice.	Fine from Rs 50/- per day.
4.	Person, who contravenes any other provision of the act.	Fine from Rs 50/- to Rs 250/

8.15 THE A.P. SHOPS & ESTABLISHMENTS RULES, 1990

INTRODUCTION

In exercise of the powers conferred by sub-section (1) of Sec. 7 I of the Andhra Pradesh Shops and Establishments Act, 1988 (Act No. 20 of 1988) the Governor of Andhra Pradesh hereby makes the Andhra Pradesh Shops & Establishments Rules as provided in the

Annexure, the same having been previously published as required by subsection (3) of Section 71 of the said Act. The said Rules shall come into force with effect from 1-11-1991.

These rules may be called the Andhra Pradesh Shops and Establishments Rules, 1990.

DEFINITIONS

1. *Act:* means the Andhra Pradesh shops and Establishments Act, 1988 ;

2. *Family members:* means father, mother, wife, husband, sons, daughters, sisters and brothers, wholly dependent on the earnings of the employer ;

3. *Form:* means a form appended to these Rules ;

REGISTRATION OF ESTABLISHMENTS AND RENEWAL OF REGISTRATION CERTIFICATE

1. The statement specified in sub-section (1) of Section 3 of the Act shall be submitted by the employer in Form-I to the Inspector of the area concerned. The statement shall be accompanied by a challan in support of the payment of fees prescribed in Schedule-I.

2. The Inspector shall maintain Register of Establishments in Form-V.

3. The Inspector shall issue a Certificate of Registration in Form-II.

4. The Inspector may, on an application made by the employer accompanied by the fees prescribed therefor, renew the registration certificate for a period of one year or for such number of years as may be prescribed, commencing from the date of its expiry. Every application for the renewal of the registration certificate shall be made in such form and in such manner as may be prescribed so as to reach the Inspector not later than thirty days before the date of its expiry.

5. The period of renewal of Certificate of Registration shall 'be one year or upto three years from the date of its expiry, at the option of the employer.

6.   On receipt of application for renewal of Certificate of Registration, the Inspector shall issue Renewal of Registration Certificate in Form IV.

7.   Where the application for Renewal of Registration Certificate is not made within the date i.e., atleast 30 days before its expiry, penalty as specified below shall be levied.

a)   Application submitted on or after 2nd December, but before 31st December: 25% of the fees Prescribed.

b)   Application submitted on or after 1st January: 50% of the fees Prescribed.

Provided that the Government or subject to the control of the Government the Chief Inspector may, if they are or he is satisfied that there is sufficient reason for the employer in not sending the application for the renewal of the Certificate of Registration before the expiry of the time limit specified in subsection (2) of Section 4, by an order and for reasons recorded therein, waive the payment of penalty either in part or wholly by the employer in respect of the renewal of the Certificate of Registration applied for.

PAYMENT OF FEES

The fees prescribed under these Rules shall be remitted into the Government Treasury/State Bank of India/ State Bank of Hyderabad under the Head of Account "0230 Labour and Employment (101) Receipts under Labour Laws". The fees once remitted shall under no circumstances be refunded.

ISSUE OF DUPLICATE REGISTRATION CERTIFICATE

If the Certificate of Registration issued under sub-rule (3) of Rule 3 is lost, destroyed or defaced, the employer of the Establishment shall forthwith report the matter to the Inspector of the area concerned and shall apply in Form-VI with a fee as prescribed in Schedule-II for the issue of duplicate registration certificate. Upon the receipt of such application together with the fee, the Inspector shall furnish to the employer with a duplicate copy of registration certificate duly stamped 'Duplicate copy of the Registration Certificate'.

NOTICE OF CHANGE

1. Notice shall be given by the employer to the Inspector of the area concerned as required under sub section (4) of Section 3 of the Act, in Form-VII together with the Certificate of Registration and a challan for the amount of fee remitted as specified in Schedule-II and the amount, if any, payable as specified in Schedule-I having regard to increase in the number of employees:

Provided that no notice need be given by the employer to the Inspector of the area concerned in respect of any change in the number of employees if such change does not affect the licence for remittance as specified in Schedule-1.

2. On receipt of notice of change the Inspector shall amend the Certificate of Registration or issue' afresh one. If necessary and send it to the employer.

3. Where the Inspector cancels the Certificate of Registration on receipt- of information with regard to the closure of Shop/ Establishment, he shall intimate the employer about the cancellation of the Registration, Certificate. The Communication to the employer shall be sent under Certificate of Posting.

AUTHORITY TO WHOM, APPEALS SHALL LIE AGAINST REVOCATION OF SUSPENSION OF REGISTRATION CERTIFLCATE

An appeal under sub-section (1) of Section 6 of the Act against the orders of revocation or suspension of the Registration Certificate shall lie to the Labour Officer in whose jurisdiction the Shop/Establishment lies.

FORM OF APPEAL, MODE OF SUBMISSION AND PROCEDURE TO BE FOLLOWED BY THE APPELLATE AUTHORITY

1. Every appeal, under Section 6 shall be presented to the Appellate Authority in person or sent to him by Registered Post under Acknowledgement Due.

2. The appeal shall be in form of, a memorandum that shall be accompanied by a certified copy of the order appealed against.

3. The memorandum shall set forth the grounds of the appeal.

4. Where the memorandum of appeal does not comply with the provisions of sub-rules (2) and (3) above, it may' be returned, within fifteen days from the date of its receipt to the appellant for the purpose of being amended. The appellant shall resubmit the appeal duly amended as directed by the Appellate Authority within a period of thirty days from the date of its return.

5. Where the memorandum of appeal is in order, the Appellate Authority shall admit the appeal, endorse thereon the date of presentation and shall register the appeal in the Register of Appeals in Form VIII.

6. Where the appeal is admitted, the Appellate Authority shall obtain the connected records from the Inspector concerned against whose order the appeal has been preferred.

7. The Appellate Authority shall give an opportunity to the appellant for being heard, by fixing a date.

8. If, on the date fixed for personal hearing, the appellant does not appear, the Appellate Authority shall decide the appeal on; the basis of the records made available to him and shall communicate his order to the appellant.

ASCERTAINMENT OF AGE BY THE INSPECTORS

An employer may be required to produce one of the following, documents in support of the age of an employee,

a) School Certificate.

b) Extract from the register of Birth.

c) Certificate in Form IX from the Government Medical Officer not below the rank of Assistant Civil Surgeon.

MATERNITY BENEFIT

1. The payment of Maternity Benefit to a woman employee under Section 25 of the Act shall be at the same rate of daily, weekly or monthly wages last paid, In the case of piece rate employees, the rate of maternity benefit shall be on the basis of the average earning of one month or wages drawn on the working day whichever is higher.

2. The payment of maternity benefit accruing to a woman employee shall be made to her at any time not later than one week after receipt of intimation in writing about the date of her delivery,

Provided that if woman dies during this period, that maternity benefit shall be payable only for the days up to and including the day of her death.

3. In case of miscarriage, the woman employee shall on production of a certificate granted to that effect by a. Registered Medical Practitioner, be entitled to the maternity benefit for a period of six weeks immediately following the date of her miscarriage.

4. The amount payable to a woman employee a maternity benefit in accordance with aforesaid rules shall, for the purpose of its recovery be deemed to be wages as defined under sub-section (23) of Section 2 of the Act.

5. Payment in respect of claim of maternity benefit shall be made by the employer to the woman employee concerned or to a person authorised by herin Writing. In the case of her death, the same shall be payable to her legal heirs.

6. No woman employee having more than two children shall be eligible for maternity benefit.

CLEANLINESS

The premises of every establishment shall be kept clean in the following manner,

1. In every establishment,

a) all the inside walls of the rooms and all the ceilings of the such rooms (whether such walls or ceilings be plastered or not) and all the passages and staircases shall be white washed or colour washed at intervals not more than two years from the time when they were last white-washed or colour washed and shall be maintained in a clean state.

b) All beams, rafters, doors, window frames and other wood work with the exception of floors shall be either whitewashed or colourwashed at intervals of not more than twelve months from the time when they were last white-washed or colour-washed or shall be painted or varnished at intervals of not more than seven years from the time when they were last painted or varnished and shall be maintained in a clean state.

2. This sub rule shall not apply to the following,

- Rooms used only for the storage of articles.

- Walls or ceilings of rooms which are made of galvanised iron, flat tiles, asbestos sheets, glazed bricks, glass slate, bamboo, thatch, cement, or polished chunam,

- Ceilings of rooms in which the lowest part is atleast 6.0 meters from the floor.

- Any other establishment or part thereof in which white-washing, colour-washing, painting or varnishing is, in the opinion of the Chief Inspector, is necessary to satisfy the requirement of Section 26 of the Act in regard to cleanliness.

3. Rubbish, filth or debris shall not be allowed to accumulate or to remain on any part of the establishment for more than 24 hours and shall be disposed of. All waste matter shall be kept in covered receptacles.

4. All drains carrying waste or sullage water or sewage shall be constructed of masonry or other impermeable material and shall be regularly flushed at least twice daily and where possible, connected with some recognised drainage line.

5.   The establishment and the compound surrounding it shall be maintained in a strictly sanitary and clean condition. The floor shall be swept or otherwise cleaned at least once daily, and the ceilings shall be dusted at least once a month.

6.   The employer shall enforce the proper use of latrines and urinals and prevent pollution by excreta or urine on the surface of the ground in the vicinity or the latrine or the urinal and the compound of the establishment. The employer shall make suitable arrangements for the regular cleaning and conserving of the latrines and urinals to the satisfaction of the Inspector.

7.   Employer shall provide drinking water and keep the area around the place of drinking water clean and properly drained.

PRECAUTIONS AGAINST FIRE

Every establishment shall provide under sub-section (I) of the Section 28 with adequate means of escape in case of fire and shall also provide water or sand and/or chemical fire extinguishers in suitable number and at suitable sites according to the nature of work carried on and the size of the premises.

SAFETY

1.   Every dangerous part of machinery in an establishment other than a shop shall be securely fenced by safeguards of substantial construction which shall be kept in position while the part of machinery is in motion or in use.

2.   In every establishment where manufacturing process is carried on with the aid of electric, power, suitable devices for disconnecting the power supply during the emergencies from running machinery shall be provided and maintained.

3.   No employee, with loose fitting clothes on, shall be allowed or made to work near the moving machinery or belt and the tight fitting clothes for the purpose shall be provided by the employer.

FIRST AID APPLIANCES

In every establishment other than a shop, a first aid box shall be kept and it shall contain the following equipment together with a book of instructions on first aid namely,

a) 3 small sterilised dressings.

b) 2 medium size sterilized dressings.

c) 2 large size sterilized dressings.

d) 2 large size sterilized burn dressings.

e) 2 (15.0 grams) packets sterilized cotton wool.

f) 1 pair of dressing scissors.

g) 1(30.0 grams) bottle containing solution of salvolatine having the dose and mode of administration indicated on the label.

h) 1(30.0 grams) bottle containing solution of iodine or mercurochrome.

i) 1 (30.0 grams) bottle containing Potassium Permanganate crystals.

j) Any antidotes for burns.

MAXIMUM PERMISSIBLE LOAD, TRAINING AND INSTRUCTION, MEDICAL EXAMINATION AND PROVISION OF TECHNICAL DEVICES

1. For the purposes of this rule, the term Regular "Manual Transport of Load" means any activity which is continuously or principally devoted to the manual transport of loads, or which normally includes, even though intermittently, the manual transport of loads.

2. The maximum permissible weight which may be transported manually by' an adult male worker shall not be more than fifty five kgs. And in the case of women and young persons the maximum permissible weight shall not be more than thirty kgs.

3. No woman employee shall be assigned to manual transport of loads during pregnancy or during the ten weeks following confinement.

4.   (i) Every employee who is assigned to manual transport of loads other than light loads shall be given, prior to such assignment, adequate training or instruction in working techniques, with a view to safeguarding health and preventing accidents.

(ii) Such training or instruction should include methods of lifting, carrying, putting down, unloading, stocking of different types of loads, and shall be given by suitably qualified persons or institutions, and be followed up, wherever practicable, by supervision on the job to ensure that the correct methods are used.

(iii) Every employee occasionally assigned to manual transport of loads shall be given appropriate instructions on the manner in which such operations may be safely carried out.

5.   (i) Every employer shall make available, suitable technical devices in order to limit or to facilitate the manual transport of loads, which shall be used.

(ii) The packaging of loads which may be transported manually should be compact and of suitable material and should as far as possible and appropriate, be equipped with devices for holding and so designed as not to create risk of injury; for example, it should not have sharp edges, projections or rough surfaces.

6.   (i) The employer shall arrange for the medical examination of fitness for employment of each employee as far as practicable and appropriate before assignment of the employees to manual transport of loads.

(ii) Medical examination shall be made every one year in respect of each such employee.

(iii) Employer shall bear the cost of medical examinations.

The training or instructions provided for in this rule shall not involve the employee in any expense.

MANNER OF CALCULATING ORDINARY RATE OF WAGES

For the purpose of the explanation of Section 37, ordinary rates of wages per hour shall be calculated by dividing the total wages payable to a person employed for the hours actually worked by him during the wage period by the number of such hours in the wage period.

Provided that hours worked by a person employed in excess of the normal daily hours during the wage period shall be excluded in calculating the number of hours actually worked by him.

DUTIES OF INSPECTORS

The Inspector shall make such inspection as may appear to him to be necessary for the purpose of satisfying himself that the provisions of the Act and of the Rules and any orders issued by the Government under the Act are duly observed. In particular, he shall satisfy himself-

a)   That the establishments are duly registered under the Act; (ii) that the registers, records and notices required to be maintained or displayed under the Act or rules are properly maintained or displayed ;

b)   That the intervals of rest and holidays required to be granted or observed under the Act or granted or observed and that the limit of hours of work and spread over laid down under the Act are not exceeded.

c)   That the provisions of the Act and any orders issued by the Government regarding the opening and closing hours are duly observed.

d)   That every employee in an establishment is furnished with a letter of appointment.

e)   That the provisions of the Act and rules regarding leave, holidays with wages' and materni1y benefit are properly observed;

f)   That the provisions of the Act and the rules relating to cleanliness, ventilation, precautions against fire and sale1y of employees are properly observed.

g)   That the provisions of the Act relating to the payment of overtime work are duly observed.

h)   That no child is allowed to work in any establishment. (2) For carrying out such inspection, the Inspector may interrogate such persons in the premises, as he may deem necessary.

Provided that no such person shall be required under this rule, to answer any question, the answer to which might tend to incriminate him.

MAINTENANCE OF REGISTERS AND RECORDS AND DISPLAY OF NOTICES

Every employer shall maintain registers and records and display notices in the following manner,

1.   Every employer shall maintain a Register of Employment in Form XXII.

2.   Every employer shall maintain a Register of Wages in Form XXIII.

3.   Every employer of an establishment other than a shop shall ' exhibit in his establishment a notice in Form XXIV specifying the day or days of the week on which his employees shall be given a holiday. The notice shall be exhibited, before the employees, to whom it relates immediately preceding the first week during which it is to have effect.

4.   Every employer shall exhibit in his establishment a notice containing such abstracts of the Act and Rules as the Government may direct.

5.   Any notice required to be exhibited under these Rules shall be exhibited in such manner that it can be readily seen and read by any person whom it affects and shall be renewed whenever becomes defaced or otherwise ceased to be clearly legible.

6.   Every employer shall maintain a Register in Form XXV for the leave granted to persons employed in his establishment.

7.   In any register or record which an employer is required to maintain under these rules, the entries relating to any day, shall be made on such date and shall be authenticated under the signature of the employer or the Manager on the same day. The entries relating to overtime work shall be made before the commencement and immediately after completion of such overtime work.

8. The registers, records and notices relating to any calendar year shall be preserved for a period of three years after the last entry is made therein.

9. Save as otherwise provided in sub, rule (4) above, all Registers, records and notices required to be maintained and exhibited shall he either in English or in the language of the majority of the employees in the establishment.

10. (a)Every employer shall maintain a Visit Book in which an Inspector visiting the establishment may record his remarks regarding any defects that may come to light at the time of his visit or give directions regarding production of any documents required to be maintained or produced under the provisions of the Act and the Rules.

(b)This Visit Book shall be bound book more or less of size (18 cm X 15 cms) containing atleast 100 pages

(c) The first page of the Visit Book shall contain the following particulars-

- Name of the Shop or Establishment.

- Address.

- Registration Number

- Name of the Employer.

- Father's Name.

- Residential Address.

(d) In case the Visit Book containing remarks passed by the Inspectors, lost, destroyed or defaced, the employer of the establishment shall report the fact forthwith in writing to the Inspector of the area and immediately arrange to maintain a new Visit Book.

(e) The Visit Book shall be kept always in the business premises of the Establishment and shall be produced or caused to be produced on demand by the Inspector.

11. Where an office, store-room, godown, warehouse or workplace used .The connection with trade and business of a shop is situated at premises other than the premises of the shop, all registers, records, Visit book and notices required to be maintained, exhibited or given under the Act of the Rules shall be separately so maintained, exhibited or given ill respect of and at such office, store, room, godown, warehouse or workplace.

12. No employer with intent to deceive shall make or cause or allow to be made, in any register, record or notice prescribed to be provided under the provisions of the Act or the Rules, an entry which is false ill any material particular, or wilfully omits or causes or allows to be omitted from any such register, record or notice; any entry which is requited to be made therein, under the provisions of the Act and Rules, or maintain or cause or allow to be maintained, more than. One set of any register, record or notice.

13. The name board of every shop or establishment shall be in Telugu and wherever other languages are used, the versions in such other languages shall be below the Telugu version.

PENALTY

Any employer who contravenes any of the provisions of these Rules shall, on conviction, be punished with a fine which may extend to fifty rupees.

For a second offence with fine which shall be not less than one hundred rupees but which may extend to two hundred rupees and for the third or subsequent offences, with a fine which shall not be less than two hundred and fifty rupees but which may extend to rupees five hundred.

PART C

FACTORIES ACT 1948

8.16 INRODUCTION

Factory Act, 1948 was passed to consolidate and amend the law regulating labour in factories. Originally the act was passed in 1948 then amended in 1950, 1951, 1954 and 1976.

Economic progress of the country and the industrial peace go hand to hand. Industrial relations are thus a vital concern of community which may be expressed in measure for the protection of its large interest.

The Factory Act extends to the whole of India. It shall come into force on the 1st day of April, 1949.

OBJECTIVES

1. To provide protection.

2. To provide the healthy, safe and hygienic conditions in the factory.

3. To take protection against risk and hazards.

4. To prevent accidents on machinery and occupational hazards.

5. To regulate and control working conditions of the workers and see welfare of the workers.

6. Provides conditions for the employment of women and young persons.

DEFINITION

1. *Adult:* Means a person who has completed his fifteenth year of age.

2. *Adolescent:* Means a person who has completed his fifteen year of age but has not completed his eighteenth year.

3. *Calendar Year:* Means the period of twelve months beginning with the first day of January in any year.

4. *Child:* means a person who has not completed his fifteenth year of age.

5.   *Competent Person:* in relation to any provision of this Act, means a person or an institution recognised as such by the Chief Inspector for the purposes of carrying out tests, examinations and inspections required to be done in a factory under the provisions of this Act having regard to-

a)   The qualifications and experience of the person and facilities available at his disposal; or

b)   The qualifications and experience of the persons employed in such institution and facilities available therein, With regard to the conduct of such tests, examinations and inspections, and more than one person or institution can be recognised as a competent person in relation to a factory.

6.   *Hazardous Process:* Means any process or activity in relation to an industry specified in the First Schedule where, unless special care is taken, raw materials used therein or the intermediate or finished products, byproducts, wastes or effluents thereof would—

a)   Cause material impairment to the health of the persons engaged in or connected therewith, or

b)   Result in the pollution of the general environment.

Provided that the State Government may, by notification in the Official Gazette, amend the First Schedule by way of addition, omission or variation of any industry specified in the said Schedule.

7.   *Young Person:* Means a person who is either a child or an adolescent.

8.   *Power:* means Electrical energy, or any other form of energy which is mechanically transmitted and is not generated by human or animal agency.

9.   *Prime Mover:* Means any engine, motor or other appliance which generates or otherwise provides power.

10.   *Transmission Machinery:* Means any shaft, wheel, drum, pulley, system of pulleys, coupling, clutch, driving belt or other appliance or device by which the motion of a prime mover is transmitted to or received by any machinery or appliance.

11. **Machinery:** Includes prime movers, transmission machinery and all other appliances whereby power is generated, transformed, transmitted or applied.

12. **Manufacturing Process:** Means any process for-

a) Making, altering, repairing, ornamenting, finishing, packing, oiling, washing, cleaning, breaking up, demolishing, or otherwise treating or adapting any article or substance with a view to its use sale, transport, delivery or disposal, or pumping oil, water, sewage or any other substance; or

b) Generating, transforming or transmitting power; or composing types for printing, printing by letter press, lithography, photogravure or other similar process or book binding; or

c) Constructing, reconstructing, repairing, refitting, finishing or breaking up ships or vessels; or

d) Preserving or storing any article in cold storage.

13. **Worker:** Means a person employed, directly or by or through any agency (including a contractor) with or without the knowledge of the principal employer, whether for remuneration or not], in any manufacturing process, or in cleaning any part of the machinery or premises used for a manufacturing process, or in any other kind of work incidental to, or connected with, the manufacturing process, or the subject of the manufacturing process but does not include any member of the armed forces of the Union;

14. **Factory:** Means any premises including the precincts thereof-

a) Whereon ten or more workers are working, or were working on any day of the preceding twelve months, and in any part of which a manufacturing process is being carried on with the aid of power, or is ordinarily so carried on, or

b) Whereon twenty or more workers are working, or were working on any day of the preceding twelve months, and in any part of which a manufacturing process is being carried on without the aid of power, or is ordinarily so carried on,- but does not include a mine subject to the operation of the Mines Act, 1952 (35 of

1952), or a mobile unit belonging to the armed forces of the Union, a railway running shed or a hotel, restaurant or eating place.

15.   Occupier: Means a person who has ultimate control over the affairs of the factory. In the case of a firm or other association of individuals, anyone of the partner or member thereof shall be deemed to be occupier. In the case government/local authority, the person appointed to manage the affairs shall be deemed to be occupier.

8.17 LICENSING PROCEDURE

Approval, Licensing and Registration of Factories

1.   The State Government may make rules-

a)   Requiring, for the purposes of this Act, the submission of plans of any class or

•   Requiring the previous permission in writing of the State Government or the Chief Inspector to be obtained for the site on which the factory is to be situated and for the construction or extension of any factory or class or description of factories;

b)   Requiring for the purpose of considering application for such permission the submission of plans and specifications;

c)   prescribing the nature of such plans and specifications and by whom they shall be certified;

d)   Requiring the registration and licensing of factories or any class or description of factories, and prescribing the fees payable for such registration and licensing and for the renewal of licences;

e)   Requiring that no licence shall be granted or renewed unless the notice specified in section 7 has been given.

2.   If on an application for permission referred to in clause (aa) of sub-section (1) accompanied by the plans and specifications required by the rules made under clause (b) of that sub-section, sent to the State Government or Chief Inspector by registered post, no order is communicated to the applicant within three months

from the date on which it is so sent, the permission applied for in the said application shall be deemed to have been granted.

3.   Where a State Government or a Chief Inspector refuses to grant permission to the site, construction or extension of a factory or to the registration and licensing of a factory, the applicant may within thirty days of the date of such refusal appeal to the Central Government if the decision appealed from was of the State Government and to the State Government in any other case.

Notice by occupier

1.   The occupier shall, at least fifteen days before he begins to occupy or use any premises as a factory, sent to the Chief Inspector a written notice containing-

a)   The name and situation of the factory.

b)   The name and address of the occupier.

●   The name and address of the owner of the premises or building (including the precincts thereof) referred to in section 93.

c)   The address to which communications relating to the factory may be sent.

d)   The nature of the manufacturing process-

●   Carried on in the factory during the last twelve months in the case of factories in existence on the date of the commencement of this Act, and

●   To be carried on in the factory during the next twelve months in the case of all factories.

e)   The total rated horse power installed or to be installed in the factory, which shall not include the rated horse power of any separate stand-by plant.

f)   The name of the manager of the factory of the purposes of this Act.

g)   The number of workers likely to be employed in the factory.

h)   The average number of workers per day employed during the last twelve months in the case of factory in existence on the date of the commencement of this Act.

- Such other particulars as may be prescribed.

2.   In respect of all establishments which come within the scope of the Act for the first time, the occupier shall send a written notice to the Chief Inspector containing the particulars specified in subsection (1) within thirty days, from the date of the commencement of this Act.

3.   Before a factory engaged in a manufacturing process which is ordinarily carried on for less than one hundred and eighty working days in the year resumes working, the occupier shall send a written notice to the Chief Inspector containing the particulars specified in sub-section (1) at least thirty days before the date of the commencement of work.

4.   Whenever a new manager is appointed, the occupier shall send to the Inspector a written notice and to the Chief Inspector a Copy Thereof within seven days from the date on which such person takes over charges.

5.   During any period for which no person has been designated as manager of a factory or during which the person designated does not manage the factory, any person found acting as manage, or if no such person is found, the occupier himself, shall be deemed to be the manager of the factory for the purposes of this Act.

8.18 HEALTH AND SAFETY

Cleanliness

1.   Every factory shall be kept clean and free from effluvia arising from any drain, privy or other nuisance, and in particular-

a)   Accumulation of dirt and refuse shall be removed daily by sweeping or by any other effective method from the floors and benches of workrooms and from staircases and passages, and disposed of in a suitable manner;

b) The floor of every workroom shall be cleaned at least once in every week by washing, using disinfectant, where necessary, or by some other effective method;

c) Where a floor is liable to become wet in the course of any manufacturing process to such extent as is capable of being drained. effective means of drainage shall be provided and maintained:

d) All inside walls and partitions, all ceilings or tops of rooms and all walls, sides and tops of passages and staircases shall-

i. Where they are painted otherwise than with washable water-paint or varnished, be repainted or revarnished at least once in every period of five years;

• Where they are painted with washable water paint, be repainted with at least one coat of such paint at least once in every period of three years and washed at least once in every period of six months;

ii. Where they are painted or varnished or where they have smooth impervious surfaces, be cleaned at least once in every period of fourteen months by such method as may be prescribed;

iii. In any other case, be kept whitewashed or colourwashes, and the whitewashing or colour washing shall be carried out at least once in every period of fourteen months;

iv. All doors and window frames and other wooden or metallic framework and shutters shall be kept painted or varnished and the painting or varnishing shall be carried out at least once in every period of five years;

e) The dates on which the processes required by clause (d) are carried out shall be entered in the prescribed register.

2. If, in view of the nature of the operations carried on in a factory or class or description of factories or any part of a factory or class or description of factories, it is not possible for the occupier to comply with all or any of the provisions of subsection (1), the State

Government may be order exempt such factory or class or description of factories or part from any of the provisions of that sub-section and specify alternative methods for keeping the factory in a clean state.

Disposal of wastes and effluents

1. Effective arrangements shall be made in every factory for the treatment of wastes and effluents due to the manufacturing process carried on therein, so as to render them innocuous and for their disposal.

2. The State Government may make rules prescribing the arrangements to be made under sub-section (1) or requiring that the arrangements made in accordance with sub-section (1) shall be approved by such authority as may be prescribed.

Ventilation and temperature

1. Effective and suitable provision shall be made in every factory for securing and maintaining in every workroom—

   a) Adequate ventilation by the circulation of fresh air, and

   b) Such a temperature as will secure to workers therein reasonable conditions of comfort and prevent injury to health; and in particular,-

   i.   Walls and roofs shall be of such material and so designed that such temperature shall not be exceeded but kept as low as practicable;

   ii.   Where the nature of the work carried on in the factory involves, or is likely to involve, the production of excessively high temperatures, such adequate measures as are practicable shall be taken to protect the workers therefrom, by separating the process which produces 'such' temperatures from the workroom, by insulating the hot parts or by other effective means.

2. The State Government may prescribe a standard of adequate ventilation and reasonable temperature for any factory or class or

description of factories or parts thereof and direct that proper measuring instruments, at such places and in such position as may be specified, shall be provided and such records, as may be prescribed, shall be maintained.

3. If it appears to the Chief Inspector that excessively high temperatures in any factory can be reduced by the adoption of suitable measures, he may, without prejudice to the rules made under subsection (2), serve on the occupier, an order in writing specifying the measures which, in his opinion, should be adopted, and requiring them to be carried out before a specified date.

Dust and fume

1. In every factory in which, by reason of the manufacturing process carried on, there is given off any dust or fume or other impurity of such a nature and to such an extent as is likely to be injurious or offensive to the workers employed therein, or any dust in substantial quantities, effective measures shall be taken to prevent its inhalation and accumulation in any workroom, and if any exhaust appliance is necessary for this purpose, it shall be applied as near as possible to the point of origin of the dust, fume or other impurity, and such point shall be enclosed so far as possible.

2. In any factory no stationary internal combustion engine shall be operated unless the exhaust is conducted into the open air, and no other internal combustion engine shall be operated in any room unless effective measures have been taken to prevent such accumulation of fumes therefrom as are likely to be injurious to workers employed in the room.

Artificial humidification

1. In respect of all factories in which the humidity of the air is artificially increased, the State Government may make rules,-

    a) Prescribing standards of humidification;

    b) Regulating the methods used for artificially increasing the humidity of the air;

c)   Directing prescribed tests for determining the humidity of the air to be correctly carried out and recorded;

d)   Prescribing methods to be adopted for securing adequate ventilation and cooling of the air in the workrooms.

2.   In any factory in which the humidity of the air is artificially increased, the water used for the purpose shall be taken from a public supply, or other source of drinking water, or shall be effectively purified before it is so used.

3.   If it appears to an Inspector that the water used in a factory for increasing humidity is required to be effectively purified under sub-section (2) is not effectively purified he may serve on the manager of the factory an order in writing, specifying the measures which in his opinion should be adopted, and requiring them to be carried out before specified date.

Overcrowding

1.   No room in any factory shall be overcrowded to an extent injurious to the health of the workers employed therein.

2.   Without prejudice to the generality of sub-section (1), there shall be in every workroom of factory in existence on the date of the commencement of this Act at least 9.9 cubic metres and of a factory built after the commencement of this Act at least 14.2 cubic meters of space for every worker employed therein, and for the purposes of this sub-section no account shall be taken of any space which is more than 4.2 meters above the level of the floor of the room.

3.   If the Chief Inspector by order in writing so requires, there shall be posted in each workroom of a factory a notice specifying the maximum number of workers who may, in compliance with the provisions of this section, be employed in the room.

4.   The chief Inspector may by order in writing exempt, subject to such conditions, if any, as he may think fit to impose, any workroom from the provisions of this section, if he is satisfied that compliance therewith in respect of the rooms is unnecessary in the interest of the health of the workers employed therein.

LIGHTING

1. In every part of a factory where workers are working or passing there shall be provided and maintained sufficient and suitable lighting, natural or artificial, or both.

2. In every factory all glazed windows and skylights used for the lighting of the workrooms shall be kept clean on both the inner and outer surfaces and, so far as compliance with the provisions of any rules made under sub-section (3) of section 13 will allow, free from obstruction.

3. In every factory effective provision shall, so far as is practicable, be made for the prevention of-

    a)   Glare, either directly from a source of light or by reflection from a smooth or polished surface;

    b)   The formation of shadows to such an extent as to cause eye-strain or the risk of accident to any worker.

4. The State Government may prescribe standards of sufficient and suitable lighting for factories or for any class of description of factories or for any manufacturing process.

DRINKING WATER

1. In every factory effective arrangements shall be made to provide and maintain at suitable points conveniently situated for all workers employed therein a sufficient supply of wholesome drinking water.

2. All such points shall be legibly marked "drinking water" in a language understood by majority of the workers employed in the factory, and no such point shall be situated within six meters of any washing place, urinal, latrine, spittoon, open drain carrying sullage or effluent or any other source of contamination unless a shorter distance is approved in writing by the Chief Inspector.

3. In every factory wherein more than two hundred and fifty workers are ordinarily employed, provision shall be made for cooling drinking water during hot weather by effective means and for distribution thereof.

4.   In respect of all factories or any class or description of factories the State Government may make rules for securing compliance with the provisions of sub-sections (1), (2) and (3) and for the examination by prescribed authorities of the supply and distribution of drinking water in factories.

LATRINES AND URINALS

1.   In every factory

a)   Sufficient latrine and urinal accommodation of prescribed types shall be provided conveniently situated and accessible to workers at all times while they at the factory;

b)   Separate enclosed accommodation shall be provided for male and female workers;

c)   Such accommodation shall be adequately lighted and ventilated, and no latrine or urinal shall, unless specially exempted in writing by the Chief Inspector, communicate with any workroom except through an intervening open space or ventilated passage;

d)   All such accommodation shall be maintained in a clean and sanitary condition at all times;

e)   Sweepers shall be employed whose primary duty it would be to keep clean latrines, urinals and washing places.

2.   In every factory wherein more than two hundred and fifty workers are ordinarily employed-

a)   All latrine and urinal accommodation shall be of prescribed sanitary types;

b)   The floors and internal walls, up to a height of ninety continents of the latrines and urinals and the sanitary blocks shall be laid in glazed tiles or otherwise finished to provided a smooth polished impervious surface;

c)   Without prejudice to the provisions of clauses (d) and (e) of sub-section (1), the floors, portions of the walls and blocks so laid or finished and the sanitary pans of latrines and urinals shall be thoroughly washed and cleaned at least once in every seven days with suitable detergents or disinfectants or with both.

3.   The State Government may prescribe the number of latrines and urinals to be provided in any factory in proportion to the numbers of male and female workers ordinarily employed therein, and provide for such further matters in respect of sanitation in factories, including the obligation of workers in this regard, as it considers necessary in the interest of the health of the workers employed therein.

SPITTOONS

1.   In every factory there shall be provided a sufficient number of spittoons in convenient places and they shall be maintained in a clean and hygienic condition.

2.   The State Government may make rules prescribing the type and the number of spittoons to be provided and their location in any factory and provide for such further matters relating to their maintenance in a clean and hygienic condition.

3.   No person shall spit within the premises of a factory except in the spittoons provided for the purposes and a notice containing this provision and the penalty for its violation shall be prominently displayed at suitable places in the premises.

4.   Whoever spits in contravention of sub-section (3) shall be punishable with fine not exceeding five rupees.

SAFETY

Fencing of machinery

1.   In every factory the following, namely,—

a)   Every moving part of a prime mover and every flywheel connected to a prime mover whether the prime mover or flywheel is in the engine house or not;

b)   The headrace and tailrace of every water-wheel and water turbine;

c)   Any part of a stock-bar which projects beyond the head stock of a lathe; and

d)   Unless they are in such position or of such construction as to be safe to every person employed in the factory as they would be if they were securely fenced, the following, namely,—

i.   Every part of an electric generator, a motor or rotary convertor;

ii.   Every part of transmission machinery; and

iii.   Every dangerous part of any other machinery, shall be securely fenced by safeguards of substantial construction which shall be constantly maintained and kept in position while the parts of machinery they are fencing are in motion or in use:

2.   The State Government may be rules prescribe such further precautions as it may consider necessary in respect of any particular machinery or part thereof, or exempt, subject to such condition as may be prescribed, for securing the safety of the workers, any particular machinery or part thereof from the provisions of this section.

Work on or near machinery in motion

1.   Where in any factory it becomes necessary to examine any part of machinery referred to in section 21, while the machinery is in motion, or, as a result of such examination, to carry out-

a)   In a case referred to in clause (i) of the proviso to sub-section (1) of section 21, lubrication or other adjusting operation; or

b)   In a case referred to in clause (ii) of the proviso aforesaid, any mounting or shipping of belts or lubrication or other adjusting operation, while the machinery is in motion, such examination or operation shall be made or carried out only by a specially trained adult male worker wearing tight fitting clothing (which shall be supplied by the occupier) whose name has been recorded in the register prescribed in this behalf and who has been furnished with a certificate of his appointment, and while he is so engaged,—

i.   Such worker shall not handle a belt at a moving pulley unless20

• The belt is not more than fifteen centimeters in width;

- The pulley is normally for the purpose of drive and not merely a fly-wheel or balance wheel (in which case a belt is not permissible);

- The belt joint is either laced or flush with the belt;

- The belt, including the joint and the pulley rim, are in good repair;

- There is reasonable clearance between the pulley and any fixed plant or structure;

- Secure foothold and, where necessary, secure handhold, are provided for the operator; and

- Any ladder in use for carrying out any examination or operation aforesaid is securely fixed or lashed or is firmly held by a second person;

ii.   Without prejudice to any other provision of this Act relating to the fencing of machinery, every set screw, bolt and key on any revolving shaft, spindle, wheel or pinion, and all spur, worm and other toothed or friction gearing in motion with which such worker would otherwise be liable to come into contact, shall be securely fenced to prevent such contact.

2. No woman or young person shall be allowed to clean, lubricate or adjust any part of a prime mover or of any transmission machinery while the prime mover or transmission machinery is in motion, or to clean, lubricate or adjust any part of any machine if the cleaning, lubrication or adjustment thereof would expose the woman or young person to risk of injury from any moving part either of that machine or of any adjacent machinery.

3. The State Government may, by notification in the Official Gazette, prohibit, in any specified factory or class or description of factories, the cleaning, lubricating or adjusting by any person of specified parts of machinery when those parts are in motion.

Safety officers

1. In every factory

a) Wherein one thousand or more workers are ordinarily employed, or

b)   Wherein, in the opinion of the State Government, any manufacturing process or operation is carried on, which process or operation involves any risk of bodily injury, poisoning or disease, or any other hazard to health, to the persons employed in the factory, the occupier shall, if so required by the State Government by notification in the Official Gazette, employ such number of Safety Officers as may be specified in that notification.

2.   The duties, qualifications and conditions of service of Safety Officers shall be such as may be prescribed by the State Government.

WELFARE

Washing facilities

1.   In every factory

a)   Adequate and suitable facilities for washing shall be provided and maintained for the use of the workers therein;

b)   Separate and adequately screened facilities shall be provided for the use of male and female workers;

c)   Such facilities shall be conveniently accessible and shall be kept clean.

2.   The State Government may, in respect of any factory or class or description of factories or of any manufacturing process, prescribe standards of adequate and suitable facilities for washing.

Facilities for storing and drying clothing

The State Government may, in respect of any factory or class or description of factories, make rules requiring the provision therein of suitable places for keeping clothing not worn during working hours and for the drying of wet clothing.

Facilities for sitting

1.   In every factory suitable arrangements for sitting shall be provided and maintained for all workers obliged to work in a standing position, in order that they may take advantage of any opportunities for rest which may occur in the course of their work.

2.   If, in, the opinion of the Chief Inspector, the workers in any factory engaged in a particular manufacturing process or working in a particular room are able to do their work efficiently in a sitting position, he may, by order in writing, require the occupier of the factory to provide before a specified date such seating arrangements as may be practicable for all workers so engaged or working.

3.   The State Government may, by notification in the Official Gazette, declare that the provisions of sub-section (1) shall not apply to any specified factory or class or description of factories or to any specified manufacturing process.

First-aid appliances

1.   There shall in every factory be provided and maintained so as to be readily accessible during all working hours first-aid boxes or cupboards equipped with the prescribed contents, and the number of such boxes or cupboards to be provided and maintained shall not be less than one for every one hundred and fifty workers ordinarily employed at any one time in the factory.

2.   Nothing except the prescribed contents shall be kept in a first-aid box or cupboard.

3.   Each first-aid box or cupboard shall be kept in the charge of a separate responsible person who holds a certificate in first-aid treatment recognised by the State Government and who shall always be readily available during the working hours of the factory.

4.   In every factory wherein more than five hundred workers are ordinarily employed there shall be provided and maintained an ambulance room of the prescribed size, containing the prescribed equipment and in the charge of such medical and nursing staff as may be prescribed and those facilities shall always be made readily available during the working hours of the factory.

Canteens

1.   The State Government may make rules requiring that in any specified factory wherein more than two hundred and fifty workers

are ordinarily employed, a canteen or canteens shall be provided and maintained by the occupier for the use of the workers.

2.   Without prejudice to the generality of the foregoing power, such rules may provide for—

a)   The date by which such canteen shall be provided;

b)   The standards in respect of construction, accommodation, furniture and other equipment of the canteen;

c)   The foodstuffs to be served therein and the charges which may be made therefor;

d)   The constitution of a managing committee for the canteen and representation of the workers in the management of the canteen;

•   The items of expenditure in the running of the canteen which are not to be taken into account in fixing the cost of foodstuffs and which shall be borne by the employer;

e)   The delegation to the Chief Inspector, subject to such conditions as may be prescribed, of the power to make rules under clause (c).

Shelters, rest rooms and lunch rooms

1.   In every factory wherein more than one hundred and fifty workers are ordinarily employed, adequate and suitable shelters or rest rooms and a suitable lunch room, with provision for drinking water, where workers can eat meals brought by them, shall be provided and maintained for the use of the workers:

Provided that any canteen maintained in accordance with the provisions of section 46 shall be regarded as part of the requirements of this subsection:

Provided further that where a lunch room exists no worker shall eat any food in the work room.

2.   The shelters or rest rooms or lunch rooms to be provided under sub-section (1) shall be sufficiently lighted and ventilated and shall be maintained in a cool and clean condition.

3.   The State Government may—

a)   Prescribe the standards in respect of construction, accommodation, furniture and other equipment of shelters, rest rooms and lunch rooms to be provided under this section;

b)   By notification in the Official Gazette, exempt any factory or class or description of factories from the requirements of this section.

Welfare officers

1.   In every factory wherein five hundred or more workers are ordinarily employed the occupier shall employ in the factory such number of welfare officers as may be prescribed.

2.   The State Government may prescribe the duties, qualifications and conditions of service of officers employed under sub-section (1).

WORKING HOURS

1.   Not more than 9hrs/day, 48hrs/week, not more than 5hrs/day at a stretch.

2.   One holiday per week.

3.   Any overtime work is entitled to wages at the rate of twice of the ordinary rate.

4.   No employee can work at two or more factories.

5.   A notice of period of work for adult worker shall be displayed.

6.   Maintain a register of adult workers.

7.   Every adult worker in a factory shall be allowed a holiday/week.

EMPLOYMENT OF WOMEN/YOUNG CHILDREN

1.   Women should be allowed to work only in between 06:00a.m to 07:00p.m.

2.   No child should be employed or allowed to work more than 4.5hrs/day and during night 10:00p.m to 06:00a.m.

LEAVES

Every worker after the completion of 240 days in a calendar year, shall allow following leaves with wages,

1.   Adult 1 day for 20 working days.

2.   Child 1 day for 15 working days.

These leaves mat be accumulated up to 30 and 40 days respectively.

SPECIAL PROVISIONS

1.   State government shall exempt public institutions (education, training or reformation) from the provisions.

2.   Notice of certain accidents: if any accident occurs which causes death or injury, the person injured may be prevented from work for 48hrs or more. The manager sh 'l send notice to the authorities.

3.   Notice of certain disease: if ant worker contracts any disease specified in schedule, manager shall send notice to authorities.

4.   Notice of certain dangerous occurrences: if any dangerous occurrence takes place in the factory which may cause bodily injury or disability, the manager of the factory shall send notice to such authorities.

5.   Enquire into accident or disease: government appoints a competent person to inquire into the cause of accident/disease.

6.   Power to take samples: the inspector may take sufficient sample to be used in the factory.

7.   Safety and occupational health survey: the proper authority may undertake safety and occupational health survey.

8.   Dangerous operation: if any operation carried on in the factory exposes any person employed into a serious risk of injury, poisoning or diseases, owner of factory should specify.

   a)   The operation and declaring it to be dangerous.

b) Prohibit or restrict the employment of women, adolescents or children in the operation.

c) Provide for periodical medical examination of person employed in the operation and prohibiting the employment of the persons not certified as fit for such employment.

d) Prohibiting, restricting or controlling the use of any specified materials or processes in connection with the operation.

OFFENCES AND PENALTIES

S.no	OFFENCES	PENALTIES
1.	Any contravention of the provision.	3 months imprisonment or Rs 2000/- fine (first conviction).
		6 months imprisonment or Rs 1000/- fine or both (second conviction).
2.	Anyone who obstrucs any inspector in the exercise of any power or donot give register or documents	3 months imprisonment or Rs 500/- fine or both.
3.	If publishes or discloses the result of analysis.	3 months imprisonment or Rs 500/- fine or both.
4.	Any worker contravenes any provision of the act.	Rs 20/- fine.
5.	If any worker uses false certificate of fitness.	1 month's imprisonment or Rs 50/- fine or both.
6.	If a child works in 2 factories at a time and his guardian obtain benefit from his wages.	Guardian punishable with Rs 50/ fine.
7.	If any worker misuses any appliances or neglects to make use of any appliances for safety.	3 months imprisonment or Rs 100/- fine or both.

PART D

GENERAL AGREEMENT ON TARIFFS AND TRADE (GATT)

8.19 INTRODUCTION

The WTO's predecessor, the GATT, was established on a provisional basis after the Second World War in the wake of other new multilateral institutions dedicated to international economic cooperation - notably the "Bretton Woods" institutions now known as the World Bank and the International Monetary Fund.

The original 23 GATT countries were among over 50 which agreed a draft Charter for an International Trade Organization (ITO) - a new specialised agency of the United Nations. The Charter was intended to provide not only world trade disciplines but also contained rules relating to employment, commodity agreements, restrictive business practices, international investment and services.

In an effort to give an early boost to trade liberalization after the Second World War - and to begin to correct the large overhang of protectionist measures which remained in place from the early 1930s - tariff negotiations were opened among the 23 founding GATT "contracting parties" in 1946. This first round of negotiations resulted in 45,000 tariff concessions affecting $10 billion - or about one-fifth - of world trade. It was also agreed that the value of these concessions should be protected by early - and largely "provisional" - acceptance of some of the trade rules in the draft ITO Charter. The tariff concessions and rules together became known as the General Agreement on Tariffs and Trade and entered into force in January 1948

Although the ITO Charter was finally agreed at a UN Conference on Trade and Employment in Havana in March 1948 ratification in national legislatures proved impossible in some cases. When the United States' government announced, in 1950, that it would not seek congressional ratification of the Havana Charter, the ITO was effectively dead. Despite its provisional nature, the GATT remained the only multilateral instrument governing international trade from 1948 until the establishment of the WTO.

Although, in its 47 years, the basic legal text of the GATT remained much as it was in 1948, there were additions in the form of "plurilateral" voluntary membership, agreements and continual efforts to reduce tariffs. Much of this was achieved through a series of "trade rounds".

TRADE ROUNDS (the package route to progress)

The biggest leaps forward in international trade liberalization have come through multilateral trade negotiations, or "trade rounds", under the auspices of GATT – the Uruguay Round was the latest and most extensive.

Although often lengthy, trade rounds offer a package approach to trade negotiations; an approach with a number of advantages over issue-by-issue negotiations. For a start, a trade round allows participants to seek and secure advantages across a wide range of issues. Second, concessions which are necessary but would otherwise be difficult to defend in domestic political terms can be made more easily in the context of a package which also contains politically and economically attractive benefits. Third, developing countries and other less powerful participants have a greater chance of influencing the multilateral system in the context of a round than if bilateral relationships between major trading nations are allowed to dominate. Finally, overall reform in politically sensitive sectors of world trade can be more feasible in the context of a global package - reform of agricultural trade was a good example in the Uruguay Round.

Most of GATT's early trade rounds were devoted to continuing the process of reducing tariffs. The results of the Kennedy Round in the mid-sixties, however, included a new GATT Anti-Dumping Agreement. The Tokyo Round during the seventies was a more sweeping attempt to extend and improve the system.

THE TOKYO ROUND (a first try at reforming the trading system)

Conducted between 1973 and 1979 and with 102 participating countries, the Tokyo Round continued GATT's efforts to progressively reduce tariffs. The results included an average one-third cut in customs duties in the world's nine major industrial markets, bringing the average tariff on manufactured products down to 4.7 per cent compared with about 40 per cent at the time of GATT's creation. The tariff reductions phased in over a period of eight years, involved an element of harmonization, bringing the highest tariffs down proportionately more than the lowest.

Elsewhere, the Tokyo Round had mixed results. It failed to come to grips with the fundamental problems affecting farm trade and also stopped short of providing a new agreement on "safeguards" (emergency import measures). Nevertheless, a series of agreements on non-tariff barriers did emerge from the negotiations, in some cases interpreting existing GATT rules, in others breaking entirely new ground. In most cases, only a relatively small number of, mainly industrialized, GATT members ascribed to these agreements and arrangements which, as a consequence, were often referred to as "codes". They include the following agreements:

Subsidies and countervailing measures - interpreting Articles VI, XVI and XXIII of the General Agreement

- Technical barriers to trade - sometimes called the Standards Code.

- Import licensing procedures.

- Government procurement.

- Customs valuation - interpreting Article VII.

- Anti-dumping- interpreting Article VI and replacing the Kennedy Round Anti-Dumping Code.

- Bovine Meat Arrangement.

- International Dairy Arrangement.

- Trade in Civil Aircraft.

Several of the above Codes were amended and extended in the Uruguay Round. Those on subsidies and countervailing measures, technical barriers to trade, import licensing, customs valuation and anti-dumping, are now multilateral commitments within the WTO Agreement -in other words, all WTO members are committed to them - while those on government procurement, bovine meat, dairy products and civil aircraft remain "plurilateral" agreements.

PROGRESS OF GATT

Given its provisional nature and limited field of action, the success of GATT in promoting and securing the liberalization of much of world trade over 47 years is incontestable. Continual reductions in tariffs alone helped spur very high rates of world trade growth - around 8 per cent a year on average - during the 1950s and1960s. And the momentum of trade liberalization helped ensure that trade growth consistently out-paced production growth throughout the GATT era. The rush of new members during the Uruguay Round demonstrated that the multilateral trading system, as then represented by GATT, was recognized as an anchor for development and an instrument of economic and trade reform.

The limited achievement of the Tokyo Round, outside the tariff reduction results, was a sign of difficult times to come. GATT's success in reducing tariffs to such a low level, combined with a series of economic recessions in the 1970s and early 1980s, drove governments to devise other forms of protection for sectors facing increased overseas competition. High rates of unemployment and constant factory closures led governments in Europe and North America to seek bilateral market-sharing arrangements with competitors and to embark on a subsidies race to maintain their holds on agricultural trade. Both these changes undermined the credibility and effectiveness of GATT.

Apart from the deterioration in the trade policy environment, it also became apparent by the early 1980s that the General Agreement was no longer as relevant to the realities of world trade as it had been in the 1940s. For a start, world trade had become far more complex and important than 40 years before: the globalization of the world economy was underway, international investment was exploding and trade in services - not covered by the rules of GATT - was of major interest to more and more countries and, at the same time, closely tied to further increases in world merchandise trade. In other respects, the GATT had been found wanting: for instance, with respect to agriculture where loopholes in the multilateral system were heavily exploited - and efforts at liberalizing agricultural trade met with little success - and in the textiles and clothing sector where an exception to the normal disciplines of GATT was negotiated in the form of the Multifibre Arrangement. Even the institutional structure of GATT and its dispute settlement system were giving cause for concern.

Together, these and other factors convinced GATT members that a new effort to reinforce and extend the multilateral system should be attempted. That effort resulted in the Uruguay Round.

THE URUGUAY ROUND (creating a new system):

The seeds of the Uruguay Round were sown in November 1982 at Ministerial Meeting of GATT members in Geneva. Although Ministers intended to launch a major new negotiation, the meeting stalled on the issue of agriculture and was widely regarded as a failure. In fact, the work programme that Ministers agreed formed the basis for what was to become the Uruguay Round negotiating agenda.

Nevertheless, it took four more years of exploring and clarifying issues and painstaking consensus -building, before Ministers met again in September 1986, in Punta del Este, Uruguay, to agree to launch the Uruguay Round. They were able to accept a negotiating agenda which covered virtually every outstanding trade policy issue including the extension of the trading system into several new areas, notably trade in services and intellectual property. It was the biggest negotiating mandate on trade ever agreed and Ministers gave themselves four years to complete it.

By 1988, the negotiations had reached the stage of a "Mid-term Review". This took the form of a Ministerial Meeting in Montreal, Canada, and led to the elaboration of the negotiating mandate for the second stage of the Round. Ministers agreed a package of early results, which included some concessions on market access for tropical products - aimed to assist developing countries - as well as a streamlined dispute settlement system and the Trade Policy Review Mechanism which provided for the first comprehensive, systematic and regular reviews of national trade policies and practices of GATT members.

At the Ministerial meeting in Brussels, in December 1990, disagreement on the nature of commitments to future agricultural trade reform led to a decision to extend the round. By December 1991, a comprehensive draft text of the "Final Act", containing legal texts fulfilling every part of the Punta del Este mandate, with the exception of market access results, was on the table in Geneva. For the following two years, the negotiations lurched continuously from impending failure to predictions of imminent success. Several deadlines came and went; farm trade was joined by services, market access, anti-dumping rules and the proposed creation of a new institution, as the major points of conflict; and differences between the United States and European Communities became central to hopes for a final, successful conclusion. It took until 15 December 1993 for every issue to be finally resolved and for negotiations on market access for goods and services to be concluded. On 15 April 1994, the deal was signed by Ministers from most of the 125 participating governments at a meeting in Marrakesh, Morocco.

WORLD TRADE ORGANISATION (WTO)

8.20 INTRODUCTION

World Trade Organization (WTO) deals with the rules of trade between nations at a global or near-global level. It's an organization for liberalizing trade. It's a forum for governments to negotiate trade agreements. It's a place for them to settle trade disputes. It operates a system of trade rules.

Essentially, the WTO is a place where member governments go, to try to sort out the trade problems they face with each other. The first step is to talk. The WTO was born out of negotiations, and everything the WTO does is the result of negotiations. The bulk of the WTO's current work comes from the 1986–94 negotiations called the Uruguay Round and earlier negotiations under the General Agreement on Tariffs and Trade (GATT). The WTO is currently the host to new negotiations, under the "Doha Development Agenda" launched in 2001.

Where countries have faced trade barriers and wanted them lowered, the negotiations have helped to liberalize trade. But the WTO is not just about liberalizing trade, and in some circumstances its rules support maintaining trade barriers.

Ex: To protect consumers or prevent the spread of disease.

WTO is a set of rules. The hearts of WTO are the WTO agreements, negotiated and signed by the bulk of the world's trading nations. These documents provide the legal ground-rules for international commerce. They are essentially contracts, binding governments to keep their trade policies within agreed limits. Although negotiated and signed by governments, the goal is to help producers of goods and services, exporters, and importers conduct their business, while allowing governments to meet social and environmental objectives.

The system's overriding purpose is to help trade flow as freely as possible so long as there are no undesirable side-effects because this is important for economic development and well-being. That partly means removing obstacles. It also means ensuring that individuals, companies and governments know what the trade rules are around the world, and giving them the confidence that there will be no sudden changes of policy. In other words, the rules have to be "transparent" and predictable.

This is a third important side to the WTO's work is to settle the disputes. Trade relations often involve conflicting interests. Agreements, including those carefully and thoroughly negotiated in the WTO system, often need interpreting. The most harmonious way to settle these differences is through some neutral procedure based on an agreed legal foundation. That is the purpose behind the dispute settlement process written into the WTO agreements.

EVOLUTION

The WTO began life on 1 January 1995, but its trading system is half a century older. Since 1948, the General Agreement on Tariffs and Trade (GATT) had provided the rules for the system. (The second WTO ministerial meeting, held in Geneva in May 1998, included a celebration of the 50th anniversary of the system.)

It did not take long for the General Agreement to give birth to an unofficial, de facto international organization, also known informally as

GATT. Over the years GATT evolved through several rounds of negotiations.

The last and largest GATT round, was the Uruguay Round which lasted from 1986 to 1994 and led to the WTO's creation. Whereas GATT had mainly dealt with trade in goods, the WTO and its agreements now cover trade in services, and in traded inventions, creations and designs (intellectual property).

PRINCIPLES OF THE TRADING SYSTEM

The WTO agreements are lengthy and complex because they are legal texts covering a wide range of activities. They deal with: agriculture, textiles and clothing, banking, telecommunications, government purchases, industrial standards and product safety, food sanitation regulations, intellectual property, and much more. But a number of simple, fundamental principles run throughout all of these documents. These principles are the foundation of the multilateral trading system.

The trading system should be,

- Without discrimination — a country should not discriminate between its trading partners (giving them equally "most favoured- nation" or MFN status); and it should not discriminate between its own and foreign products, services or nationals (giving them "national treatment");

- Free — barriers coming down through negotiation;

- Predictable — foreign companies, investors and governments should be confident that trade barriers (including tariffs and non-tariff barriers) should not be raised arbitrarily; tariff rates and market-opening commitments are "bound" in the WTO;

- More competitive — discouraging "unfair" practices such as export subsidies and dumping products at below cost to gain market share;

- More beneficial for less developed countries— giving them more time to adjust, greater flexibility, and special privileges.

8.21 DIFFERENCE BETWEEN WTO AND GATT

The World Trade Organization is not a simple extension of GATT; on the contrary, it completely replaces its predecessor and has a very different character. Among the principal differences are the following:

The GATT was a set of rules, a multilateral agreement, with no institutional foundation, only a small associated secretariat, which had its origins in the attempt to establish an International Trade Organization in the 1940s. The WTO is a permanent institution with its own secretariat.

The GATT was applied on a "provisional basis" even if, after more than forty years, governments chose to treat it as a permanent commitment. The WTO commitments are full and permanent.

The GATT rules applied to trade in merchandise goods. In addition to goods, the WTO covers trade in services and trade-related aspects of intellectual property.

While GATT was a multilateral instrument, by the 1980s many new agreements had been added of a plurilateral, and therefore selective, nature. The agreements, which constitute the WTO, are almost all multilateral and, thus, involve commitments for the entire membership.

The WTO dispute settlement system is faster, more automatic, and thus much less susceptible to blockages, than the old GATT system. The implementation of WTO dispute findings will also be more easily assured.

The "GATT 1947" will continue to exist until the end of 1995, thereby allowing all GATT member countries to accede to the WTO and permitting an overlap of activity in areas like dispute settlement. Moreover, GATT lives on as "GATT 1994", the amended and up-dated version of GATT 1947, which is an integral part of the WTO Agreement and which continues to provide the key disciplines affecting international trade in goods.

THE PATENTS ACT- 1970

8.22 INRODUCTION

1. This Act may be called the Patents Act, 1970.

2. It extends to the whole of India.

3. It shall come into force on such date as the Central Government may, by notification in the Official Gazette, appoint:

Provided that different dates may be appointed for different provisions of this Act, and any reference in any such provision to the commencement of this Act shall be construed as a reference to the coming into force of that provision.

DEFINITION:

1. *Assignee:* includes the legal representative of a deceased assignee and references to the assignee of the legal representative or assignee of that person;

2. *Controller:* means the Controller General of Patents, Designs and Trade Marks referred to in section 73;

3. *Convention Application:* Means an application for a patent made by virtue of section 135;

4. *Convention country:* Means a country notified as such under sub section (1) of Section 133;

5. *Exclusive licence:* Means a licence from a patentee which confers on the licensee, or on the licensee and persons authorised by him, to the exclusion of all other persons (including the patentee), any right in respect of the patented invention, and "exclusive licensee" shall be construed accordingly:

6. *Invention:* Means any new and useful-art, process, method or manner of manufacture;

    a) machine, apparatus or other article;

    b) substance produced by manufacture,

and includes any new and useful improvement of any of them, and an alleged invention.

7. **_Legal representative:_** Means a person who in law represents the estate of a deceased person;

8. **_Medicine or drug:_** Includes-

   a)   all medicines for internal or external use of human beings or animals,

   b)   all substances intended to be used for or in the diagnosis, treatment, mitigation or prevention of diseases in human beings or animals,

   c)   all substances intended to be used or in the maintenance of public health, or the prevention or control of any epidemic disease among human beings or animals,

   d)   insecticides, germicides, fungicides, weedicides and all other substances intended to be used for the protection or preservation of plants,

   e).   all chemical substances which are ordinarily used as intermediates in the preparation or manufacture of any of the medicines or substances above referred to;

9. **_Patent:_** Means a patent granted under this Act and includes for the purposes of sections 44, 49, 50, 51, 52, 54, 55, 56, 57, 58, 63, 65, 66, 68, 69, 70, 78, 134, 140, 153, 154, and 156 and Chapters XVI, XVII and XVIII, a patent granted under the Indian Patents and Designs Act, 1911;

10. **_Patent agent:_** Means a person for the time being registered under this Act as a patent agent;

11. **_Patented article and Patented process:_** Mean respectively an article or process in respect of which a patent is in force;

12. **_Patentee:_** Means the person for the time being entered on the register as the grantee or proprietor of the patent;

13. ***True and First inventor:*** Does not include either the first importer of an invention into India, or a person to whom an invention is first communicated from outside India.

INVENTIONS NOT PATENTABLE

The following are not inventions within the meaning of this Act, -

1. An invention which is frivolous or which claims anything obvious contrary to well established natural laws;

2. An invention the primary or intended use of which would be contrary to law or morality or injurious to public health;

3. The mere discovery of a scientific principle or the formulation of an abstract theory;

4. The mere discovery of any new property of new use for a known substance or of the mere use of a known process, machine or apparatus unless such known process results in a new product or employs at least one new reactant;

5. A substance obtained by a mere admixture resulting only in the aggregation of the properties of the components thereof or a process for producing such substance;

6. The mere arrangement or re-arrangement or duplication of known devices each functioning independently of one another in a known way;

7. A method or process of testing applicable during the process of manufacture for rendering the machine, apparatus or other equipment more efficient or for the improvement or restoration of the existing machine, apparatus or other equipment or for the improvement or control of manufacture;

8. A method of agriculture or horticulture;

9. Any process for the medicinal, surgical, curative, prophylactic or other treatment of human beings or any process for a similar treatment of animals or plants to render them free of disease or to increase their economic value or that of their products.

Inventions relating to atomic energy not patentable:

No patent shall be granted in respect of an invention relating to atomic energy falling within sub-section (1) of Section 20 of the Atomic Energy Act, 1962. 33 of 1962.

Inventions where only methods or processes of manufacture patentable

1.   In the case of inventions-

a.   Claiming substances intended for use, or capable of being used, as food or as medicine or drug, or

b.   Relating to substances prepared or produced by chemical processes (including alloys, optical glass, semi-conductors and inter-metallic compounds), no patent shall be granted in respect of claims for the substances themselves, but claims for the methods or processes of manufacture shall be patentable.

2.   Notwithstanding anything contained in sub-section (1), a claim for patent of an invention for a substance itself intended for use, or capable of being used, as medicine or drug, except the medicine or drug specified under sub-clause (v) of clause (1) of sub-section (1) of section 2, may be made and shall be dealt, without prejudice to the other provisions of this Act.

8.23 APPLICATIONS FOR PATENTS

Persons entitled to apply for patents

1.   Subject to the provisions contained in section 134, an application for a patent for an invention may be made by any of the following persons, that is to say, -

a.   By any person claiming to be the true and first inventor of the invention;

b.   By any person being the assignee of the person claiming to be the true and first inventor in respect of the right to make such an application;

c.   By the legal representative of any deceased person who immediately before his death was entitled to make such an application.

2.   An application under sub-section (1) may be made by any of the persons preferred to therein either alone or jointly with any other person.

Form of application

1.   Every application for a patent shall be for one invention only and shall be made in the prescribed form and filed in the patent office.

2.   Where the application is made by virtue of an assignment of the right to apply for a patent for the invention, there shall be furnished with the application, or within such period as may be prescribed after the filing of the application, proof of the right to make the application.

3.   Every application under this section shall state that the applicant is in possession of the invention and shall name the owner claiming to be the true and first inventor; and where the person so claiming is not the applicant or one of the applicants, the application shall contain a declaration that the applicant believes the person so named to be the true and first inventor.

4.   Every such application (not being a convention application) shall be accompanied by a provisional or a complete specification.

Information and undertaking regarding foreign applications

1.   Where an applicant for a patent under this Act is prosecuting either alone or jointly with any other person an application for a patent in any country outside India in respect of the same or substantially the same invention, or where to his knowledge such an application is being prosecuted by some person through whom he claims or by some person deriving title from him, he shall file along with his application -

a.   A statement setting out the name of the country where the application is being prosecuted, the serial number and date of filing of the application and such other particulars as may be prescribed; and

b.   An undertaking that, up to the date of the acceptance of his complete specification filed in India, he would keep the Controller informed in writing, from time to time, of details of the nature referred to in clause (a) in respect of every other application relating to the same or substantially the same invention, if any, filed in any country outside India subsequently to the filing of the statement referred to in the aforesaid clause, within the prescribed time.

2.   The Controller may also require the applicant to furnish, as far as may be available to the applicant, details relating to the objections, if any, taken to any such application as is referred to in sub-section (1) on the ground that the invention is lacking in novelty or patentability, the amendments effected in the specifications, the claims allowed in respect thereof and such other particulars as he may require.

Provisional and complete specifications

1.   Where an application for a patent (not being a convention application) is accompanied by a provisional specification, a complete specification shall be filed within twelve months from the date of filing of the application, and if the complete specification is not so filed the application shall be deemed to be abandoned:

Provided that the complete specification may be filed at any time after twelve months but within fifteen months from the date aforesaid, if a request to that effect is made to the Controller and the prescribed fee is paid on or before the date on which the complete specification is filed.

2.   Where two or more applications in the name of the same applicant are accompanied by provisional specifications in respect of inventions which are cognate or of which one is a modification of another and the Controller is of opinion that the whole of such inventions are such as to constitute a single invention and may properly be included in one patent, he may allow one complete specification to be filed in respect of all such provisional specifications.

3. Where an application for a patent (not being a convention application) is accompanied by a specification purporting to be a complete specification, the Controller may, if the applicant so requests at any time before the acceptance of the specification, direct that such specification shall be treated for the purposes of this Act as a provisional specification and proceed with the application accordingly.

4. Where a complete specification has been filed in pursuance of an application for a patent accompanied by a provisional specification or by a specification treated by virtue of a direction under sub-section (3) as a provisional specification, the Controller may, if the applicant so requests at any time before the acceptance of the complete specification, cancel the provisional specification and post-date the application to the date of filing of the complete specification.

Contents of specifications

1. Every specification, whether provisional or complete, shall describe the invention and shall begin with a title sufficiently indicating the subject-matter to which the invention relates.

2. Subject to any rules that may be made in this behalf under this Act, drawings may, and shall, if the Controller so requires, be supplied for the purposes of any specification, whether complete or provisional; and any drawings so supplied shall, unless the Controller otherwise directs, be deemed to form part of the specification, and references in this Act to a specification shall be construed accordingly.

3. If, in any particular case, the Controller considers that an application should be further supplemented by a model or sample of anything illustrating the invention or alleged to constitute an invention, such model or sample as he may require shall be furnished before the acceptance of the application, but such model or sample shall not be deemed to form part of the specification.

4. Every complete specification shall-

a. Fully and particularly describe the invention and its operation or use and the method by which it is to be performed;

b.   Disclose the best method of performing the invention which is known to the applicant and for which he is entitled to claim protection; and

c.   End with a claim or claims defining the scope of the invention for which protection is claimed.

5.   The claim or claims of a complete specification shall relate to a single invention, shall be clear and succinct and shall be fairly based on the matter disclosed in the specification and shall, in the case of an invention such as is referred to in section 5, relate to a single method or process of manufacture.

6.   A declaration as to the inventorship of the invention shall, in such cases as may be prescribed, be furnished in the prescribed form with the complete specification or within such period as may be prescribed after the filing of that specification.

7.   Subject to the foregoing provisions of this section, a complete specification filed after a provisional specification may include claims in respect of developments of, or additions to, the invention which was described in the provisional specification, being developments or additions in respect of which the applicant would be entitled under the provisions of section 6 to make a separate application for a patent.

Priority dates of claims of a complete specification

1.   There shall be a priority date for each claim of a complete specification.

2.   Where a complete specification is filed in pursuance of a single application accompanied by -

a.   A provisional specification; or

b.   A specification which is treated by virtue of a direction under sub-section (3) of section 9 as a provisional specification, and the claim is fairly based on the matter disclosed in the specification referred to in clause (a) or clause (b), the priority date of that claim shall be the date of the filing of the relevant specification.

3. Where the complete specification is filed or proceeded with in pursuance of two or more applications accompanied by such specifications as are mentioned in sub-section (2) and the claim is fairly based on the matter disclosed -

    a.   In one of those specifications, the priority date of that claim shall be the date of the filing of the application accompanied by that specification;

    b.   Partly in one and partly in another, the priority date of that claim shall be the date of the filing of the application accompanied by the specification of the later date.

4. Where the complete specification has been filed in pursuance of a further application made by virtue of sub-section (1) of section 16 and the claim is fairly based on the matter disclosed in any of the earlier specifications, provisional or complete, as the case may be, the priority date of that claim shall be the date of the filing of that specification in which the matter was first disclosed.

5. Where, under the foregoing provisions of this section, any claim of a complete specification would, but for the provisions of this sub-section, have two or more priority dates, the priority date of that claim shall be the earlier or earliest of those dates.

6. In any case to which sub-sections (2), (3), (4) and (5) do not apply, the priority date of a claim shall, subject to the provisions of section 137, be the date of filing of the complete specification.

7. The reference to the date of the filing of the application or of the complete specification in this section shall, in cases where there has been a post-dating under section 9 or section 17 or, as the case may be, an ante-dating under section 16, be a reference to the date as so post-dated or ante-dated.

8. A claim in a complete specification of a patent shall not be invalid by reason only of -

    a.   The publication or use of the invention so far as claimed in that claim on or after the priority date of such claim; or

b.   The grant of another patent which claims the invention, so far as claimed in the first mentioned claim, in a claim of the same or a later priority date.

8.24 EXAMINATION OF APPLICATIONS

Examination of application

1.   When the complete specification has been led in respect of an application for a patent, the application and the specification relating thereto shall be referred by the Controller to an Examiner for making a report to him in respect of the following matters, namely:-

a.   Whether the application and the specification relating thereto are in accordance with the requirements of this Act and of any rules made thereunder;

b.   Whether there is any lawful ground of objection to the grant of the patent under this Act in pursuance of the application;

c.   The result of investigations made under section 13; and

d.   Any other matter which may be prescribed.

2.   The Examiner to whom the application and the specification relating thereto are referred under sub-section (1) shall ordinarily make the report to the Controller within a period of eighteen months from the date of such reference.

Search for Anticipation by previous publication and by prior claim

1.   The Examiner to whom an application for a patent is referred under section 12 shall make investigation for the purpose of ascertaining whether the invention so far as claimed in any claim of the complete specification -

a.   Has been anticipated by publication before the date of filing of the applicant's complete specification in any specification filed in pursuance of an application for a patent made in India and dated on or after the 1st day of January, 1912;

b.   Is claimed in any claim of any other complete specification published on or after the date of filing of the applicant's complete specification, being a specification filed in pursuance of an application for a patent made in India and dated before or claiming the priority date earlier than that date.

2. The Examiner shall, in addition, make such investigation as the Controller may direct for the purpose of ascertaining whether the invention, so far as claimed in any claim of the complete specification, has been anticipated by publication in India or elsewhere in any document other than those mentioned in sub-section (1) before the date of filing of the applicant's complete specification.

3. Where a complete specification is amended under the provisions of this Act before it has been accepted, the amended specification shall be examined and investigated in like manner as the original specification.

4. The examination and investigations required under section 12 and this section shall not be deemed in any way to warrant the validity of any patent, and no liability shall be incurred by the Central Government or any officer thereof by reason of, or in connection with, any such examination or investigation or any report or other proceedings consequent thereon.

Consideration of Report of examiner by Controller

Where, in respect of an application for a patent, the report of the Examiner received by the Controller is adverse to the applicant or requires any amendment of the application or of the specification to ensure compliance with the provisions of this Act or of the rules made thereunder, the Controller, before proceeding to dispose of the application in accordance with the provisions hereinafter appearing, shall communicate the gist of the objections to the applicant and shall, if so required by the applicant within the prescribed time, give him an opportunity of being heard.

Power of Controller to refuse or require amended applications in certain cases

1. Where the Controller is satisfied that the application or any specification filed in pursuance thereof does not comply with the

requirements of this Act or of any rules made thereunder, the Controller may either -

a.   Refuse to proceed with the application; or

b.   Require the application, specification or drawings to be amended to his satisfaction before he proceeds with the application.

2.   If it appears to the Controller that the invention claimed in the specification is not an invention within the meaning of, or is not patentable under, this Act, he shall refuse the application.

3.   If it appears to the Controller that any invention, in respect of which an application for a patent is made, might be used in any manner contrary to law, he may refuse the application, unless the specification is amended by the insertion of such disclaimer in respect of that use of the invention, or such other reference to the illegality thereof, as the Controller thinks fit.

Power of Controller to make orders respecting division of application

1.   A person who has made an application for a patent under this Act may, at any time before the acceptance of the complete specification, if he so desires, or with a view to remedy the objection raised by the Controller on the ground that the claims of the complete specification relate to more than one invention, file a further application in respect of an invention disclosed in the provisional or complete specification already filed in respect of the first mentioned application.

2.   The further application under sub-section (1) shall be accompanied by a complete specification, but such complete specification shall not include any matter not in substance disclosed in the complete specification filed in pursuance of the first mentioned application.

3.   The Controller may require such amendment of the complete specification filed in pursuance of either the original or the further application as may be necessary to ensure that neither of the said complete specifications includes a claim for any matter claimed in the other.

Power of Controller to make order respecting dating of application

1. Subject to the provisions of section 9, at any time after the filing of an application and before acceptance of the complete specification under this Act, the Controller may, at the request of the applicant made in the prescribed manner, direct that the application shall be post-dated to such date as may be specified in the request, and proceed with the application accordingly :

   Provided that no application shall be post-dated under this sub-section to a date later than six months from the date on which it was actually made or would, but for the provisions of this sub-section, be deemed to have been made.

2. Where an application or specification (including drawings) is required to be amended under clause (b) of sub-section (1) of section 15, the application or specification shall, if the Controller so directs, be deemed to have been made on the date on which the requirement is complied with or where the application or specification is returned to the applicant, on the date on which it is re-filed after complying with the requirement.

Power of Controller in cases of anticipation

1. Where it appears to the Controller that the invention so far as claimed in any claim of the complete specification has been anticipated in the manner referred to in clause (a) of sub-section (1) or sub-section (2) of section 13, he may refuse to accept the complete specification unless the applicant -

   a. Shows to the satisfaction of the Controller that the priority date of the claim of his complete specification is not later than the date on which the relevant document was published; or

   b. Amends his complete specification to the satisfaction of the Controller.

2. If it appears to the Controller that the invention is claimed in a claim of any other complete specification referred to in clause (b) of sub-section (1) of section 13, he may, subject to the provisions hereinafter contained, direct that a reference to that other

specification shall be inserted by way of notice to the public in the applicant's complete specification unless within such time as may be prescribed, -

a.   The applicant shows to the satisfaction of the Controller that the priority date of his claim is not later than the priority date of the claim of the said other specification; or

b.   The complete specification is amended to the satisfaction of the Controller.

3.   If it appears to the Controller, as a result of an investigation under section 13 or otherwise, -

a.   That the invention so far as claimed in any claim of the applicant's complete specification has been claimed in any other complete specification referred to in clause (a) of sub-section (1) of section 13; and

b.   That such other complete specification was published on or after the priority date of the applicant's claim, then, unless it is shown to the satisfaction of the Controller that the priority date of the applicant's claim is not later than the priority date of the claim of that specification, the provisions of sub-section (2) shall apply thereto in the same manner as they apply to a specification published on or after the date of filing of the applicant's complete specification.

4.   Any order of the Controller under sub-section (2) or sub-section (3) directing the insertion of a reference to another complete specification shall be of no effect unless and until the other patent is granted.

Powers of Controller in case of potential infringement.

1.   If, in consequence of the investigations required by the foregoing provisions of this Act or of proceedings under section 25, it appears to the Controller that an invention in respect of which an application for a patent has been made cannot be performed without substantial risk of infringement of a claim of any other patent, he may direct that a reference to that other patent shall be inserted in the applicant's

complete specification by way of notice to the public, unless within such time as may be prescribed -

a.   The applicant shows to the satisfaction of the Controller that there are reasonable grounds for contesting the validity of the said claim of the other patent; or

b.   The complete specification is amended to the satisfaction of the Controller.

2.   Where, after a reference to another patent has been inserted in a complete specification in pursuance of a direction under sub-section (1) -

a.   That other patent is revoked or otherwise ceases to be in force; or

b.   The specification of that other patent is amended by the deletion of the relevant claim; or

c.   It is found, in proceedings before the court or the Controller, that the relevant claim of that other patent is invalid or is not infringed by any working of the applicant's invention, the Controller may, on the application of the applicant, delete the reference to that other patent.

Powers of Controller to make orders regarding substitution of applicants, etc

1.   If the Controller is satisfied, on a claim made in the prescribed manner at any time before a patent has been granted, that by virtue of any assignment or agreement in writing made by the applicant or one of the applicants for the patent or by operation of law, the claimant would, if the patent were then granted, be entitled thereto or to the interest of the applicant therein, or to an undivided share of the patent or of that interest, the Controller may, subject to the provisions of this section, direct that the application shall proceed in the name of the claimant or in the names of the claimants and the applicant or the other joint applicant or applicants, accordingly as the case may require.

2.   No such direction as aforesaid shall be given by virtue of any assignment or agreement made by one of two or more joint applicants for a patent except with the consent of the other joint applicant or applicants.

3.   No such direction as aforesaid shall be given by virtue of any assignment or agreement for the assignment of the benefit of an invention unless -

a.   The invention is identified therein by reference to the number of the application for the patent; or

b.   There is produced to the Controller an acknowledgement by the person by whom the assignment or agreement was made that the assignment or agreement relates to the invention in respect of which that application is made; or

c.   The rights of the claimant in respect of the invention have been finally established by the decision of a court; or

d.   The Controller gives directions for enabling the application to proceed or for regulating the manner in which it should be proceeded with under sub-section (5).

4.   Where one of two or more joint applicants for a patent dies at any time before the patent has been granted, the Controller may, upon a request in that behalf made by the survivor or survivors, and with the consent of the legal representative of the deceased, direct that the application shall proceed in the name of the survivor or survivors alone.

5.   If any dispute arises between joint applicants for a patent whether or in what manner the application should be proceeded with, the Controller, may upon application made to him in the prescribed manner by any of the parties, and after giving to all parties concerned an opportunity to be heard, give such directions as he thinks fit for enabling the application to proceed in the name of one or more of the parties alone or for regulating the manner in which it should be proceeded with, or for both those purposes, as the case may require.

Time for putting application in order for acceptance

1. An application for a patent shall be deemed to have been abandoned unless within fifteen months from the date on which the first statement of objections to the application or complete specification is forwarded by the Controller to the applicant or within such longer period as may be allowed under the following provisions of this section the applicant has complied with all the requirements imposed on him by or under this Act, whether in connection with the complete specification or otherwise in relation to the application.

2. The period of fifteen months specified in sub-section (1) shall, on request made by the applicant in the prescribed manner and before the expiration of the period so specified, be extended for a further period so requested (hereafter in this section referred to as the extended period), so, however, that the total period for complying with the requirements of the Controller does not exceed eighteen months from the date on which the objections referred to in sub-section (1) are forwarded to the applicant.

3. If at the expiration of the period of fifteen months specified in sub-section (1) or the extended period -

   a.   An appeal to the High Court is pending in respect of the application for the patent for the main invention, or

   b.   In the case of an application for a patent of addition, an appeal to the High Court is pending in respect of either that application or the application for the main invention, the time within which the requirements of the Controller shall be complied with shall, on an application made by the applicant before the expiration of the said period of fifteen months or the extended period, as the case may be, be extended until such date as the High Court may determine.

4. If the time within which the appeal mentioned in sub-section (3) may be instituted has not expired, the Controller may extend the period of fifteen months, or as the case may be, the extended period, until the expiration of such further period as he may determine:

Provided that if an appeal has been filed during the said further period, and the High Court has granted any extension of time for complying with, the requirements of the Controller, then, the requirements may be complied with within the time granted by the Court.

Acceptance of complete specification

Subject to the provisions of section 21, the complete specification filed in pursuance of an application for a patent may be accepted by the Controller at any time after the applicant has complied with the requirements mentioned in sub-section (1) of that section, and, if not so accepted within the period allowed under that section for compliance with those requirements, shall be accepted as soon as may be thereafter:

Provided that the applicant may make an application to the Controller in the prescribed manner requesting him to postpone acceptance until such date [not being later than eighteen months from the date on which the objections referred to in sub-section (1) of section 21 are forwarded to the applicant] as may be specified in the application, and, if such application is made, the Controller may postpone acceptance accordingly.

Advertisement of acceptance of complete specification

On the acceptance of a complete specification, the Controller shall give notice thereof to the applicant and shall advertise in the Official Gazette the fact that the specification has been accepted, and thereupon the application and the specification with the drawings (if any) filed in pursuance thereof shall be open to public inspection.

Effect of acceptance of complete specification

On and from the date of advertisement of the acceptance of a complete specification and until the date of sealing of a patent in respect thereof, the applicant shall have the like privileges and rights as if a patent for the invention had been sealed on the date of advertisement of acceptance of the complete specification:

Provided that the applicant shall not be entitled to institute any proceedings for infringement until the patent has been sealed.

8.25 EXCLUSIVE MARKETING RIGHTS

Application for grant of exclusive rights

1. Notwithstanding anything contained in sub-section (1) of section 12, the Controller shall not, under that sub-section, refer an application in respect of a claim for a patent covered under sub-section (2) of section 5 to an Examiner for making a report till the 31st day of December, 2004 and shall, where an application for grant of exclusive right to sell or distribute the article or substance in India has been made in the prescribed form and manner and on payment of prescribed fee, refer the application for patent, to an Examiner for making a report to him as to whether the invention is not an invention within the meaning of this Act in terms of section 3 or the invention is an invention for which no patent can be granted in terms of section 4.

2. Where the Controller, on receipt of a report under sub-section (1) and after such other investigation as he may deed necessary, is satisfied that the invention is not an invention within the meaning of this Act in terms of section 3 or the invention is an invention for which no patent can be granted in terms of section 4, he shall reject the application for exclusive right to sell or distribute the article or substance.

3. In a case where an application for exclusive right to sell or distribute an article or a substance is not rejected by the Controller on receipt of a report under sub-section (1) and after such other investigation, if any, made by him, he may proceed to grant exclusive right to sell or distribute the article or substance in the manner provided in section 24B.

Grant of exclusive of rights

1. Where a claim for patent covered under sub-section 2 of section 5 has been made and the applicant has –

a. where an invention has been made whether in India or a country other than India and before filing search a claim, filed an application for the same invention claiming identical article or substance in a convention country on or after the Ist day of January, 1995 and the patent and the approval to sell or distribute the article or substance on the basis of appropriate tests conducted on or after the Ist day of January, 1995 in that country has been granted or after the date of making claim for patent covered under sub-section 2 of section 5; or

b.   where an invention has been made in India and before filing search a claim, made a claim for patent on or after the Ist day of January, 1995 for method or a process of manufacture for that invention relating to identical article or substance and has been granted in India the patent therefor on or after the making the claim for patent covered under sub-section 2 of section 5, and has been received the approval to sell or distribute the article or substance from the authority specify in this behalf by the Central Government, then, we shall have the exclusive right by himself, his agents or licencee to sell or distribute in India the article or the substance on or from the date of approval granted by the Controller in this behalf till a period of five years or till the date of grant of patent or the date of rejection of application for the grant of patent, whichever is earlier.

PART E

PHARMACEUTICAL POLICY 2002

8.26 INTRODUCTION

1. The basic objectives of governments Policy relating to the drugs and pharmaceutical sector were enumerated in the Drug Policy of 1986. These basic objectives still remain largely valid. However, the drug and pharmaceutical industry in the country today faces 26new challenges on account of liberalization of the Indian economy, the globalization of the world economy and on account of new obligations undertakenby India under the WTO Agreements. These challenges require a change in emphasis in the current pharmaceutical policy and the need for new initiatives beyond those enumerated in the Drug Policy 1986, as modified in 1994, so that policy inputs are directed more towards promoting more internationally competitive. The need for radically improving the policy framework for knowledge-based industry has also been acknowledged by the Government. The Prime Minister's Advisory Council on Trade and Industry has made important recommendations regarding knowledge-based industry. The pharmaceutical industry has been identified as one of the most important knowledge -based industries in which India has a comparative advantage.

2. The process of liberalization set in motion in 1991 has considerably reduced the scope of industrial licensing and demolished many non-tariff barriers to imports. Important steps already taken in this regard are: -

   a) Industrial licensing for the manufacture of all drugs and pharmaceuticals has been abolished except for bulk drugs produced by the use of recombinant DNA technology, bulk drugs requiring in-vivo use of nucleic acids, and specific cell/tissue targeted formulations.

b)   Reservation of 5 drugs for manufacture by the public sector only was abolished in Feb. 1999, thus opening them up for manufacture by the private sector also.

c)   Foreign investment through automatic route was raised from 51% to 74% in March 2000 and the same has been raised to 100%.

d)   Automatic approval for Foreign Technology Agreements is being given in the case of all bulk drugs, their intermediates and formulations except those produced by the use of recombinant DNA technology, for which the procedure prescribed by the Government would be followed.

e)   Drugs and pharmaceuticals manufacturing units in the public sector are being allowed to face competition including competition from imports. Wherever possible, these units are being privatized.

f)   Extending the facility of weighted deductions of 150% of the expenditure on in-house research and development to cover as eligible expenditure, the expenditure on filing patents, obtaining regulatory approvals and clinical trials besides R&D in biotechnology.

g)   Introduction of the Patents (Second Amendment) bill in the Parliament. It, inter-alia, provides for the extension in the life of a patent to 20 years.

3.   The impact of the policies enunciated, from time to time, by the government has been salutary. It has enabled the pharmaceutical industry to meet almost entirely the country's demand for formulations and substantially for bulk drugs. In the process the pharmaceutical industry in India has achieved global recognition as a low cost producer and supplier of quality bulk drugs and formulations to the world. In 1999-2000, drugs and pharmaceutical exports were Rs.6631 crores out of a total production of Rs.19,737 crores. However, two major issues have surfaced on account of globalization and implementation of our obligations under TRIP's which impact on long-term competitiveness of Indian industry. These have been addressed in the Pharmaceutical Policy -2002.

A reorientation of the objectives of the current policy has also become necessary on account of these issues:-

a)   The essentiality of improving incentives for research and development in the Indian pharmaceutical industry, to enable the industry to achieve sustainable growth particularly in view of anticipated changes in the Patent Law, and

b)   The need for reducing further the rigours of price control particularly in view of the ongoing process of liberalization.

4.   It is against this backdrop, that Pharmaceutical Policy-2002 is being enunciated.

OBJECTIVES

The main objectives of this policy are: -

1.   Ensuring abundant availability at reasonable prices within the country of good quality essential pharmaceuticals of mass consumption.

2.   Strengthening the indigenous capability for cost effective quality production and exports of pharmaceuticals by reducing barriers to trade in the pharmaceutical sector.

3.   Strengthening the system of quality control over drug and pharmaceutical production and distribution to make quality an essential attribute of the Indian pharmaceutical industry and promoting rational use of pharmaceuticals.

4.   Encouraging R&D in the pharmaceutical sector in a manner compatible with the country's needs and with particular focus on diseases endemic or relevant to India by creating an environment conducive to channelizing a higher level of investment into R&D in pharmaceuticals in India.

5.   Creating an incentive framework for the pharmaceutical industry which promotes new investment into pharmaceutical industry and encourages the introduction of new technologies and new drugs.

APPROACH ADOPTED IN THE REVIEW

1.   In order to strengthen the pharmaceutical industry's research and development capabilities and to identify the support required by Indian pharmaceutical companies to undertake domestic R&D, a Committee was set up in 1999 by this Department by the name of Pharmaceutical Research and Development Committee (PRDC) under the Chairmanship of Director General of CSIR.

2.   To qualify as R&D intensive company in India the PRDC has suggested following conditions (gold standards): -

a)   Invest at least 5% of its turnover per annum in R&D.

b)   Invest at least Rs.10 Crore per annum in innovative research including new drug development, new delivery systems etc. in India.

c)   Employ at least 100 research scientists in R&D in India.

d)   Has been granted at least 10 patents for research done in India.

e)   Own and operate manufacturing facilities in India.

3.   The recommendations of the PRDC in so far as they relate to the Pharmaceutical Policy have been taken into account while formulating the proposals on pricing aspects.

4.   The Pharmaceutical Research & Development committee has recommended in its report, submitted interalia, the setting up of a Drug Development Promotion Foundation (DDPF) and a Pharmaceutical Research & Development Support Fund (PRDSF). Necessary action in this regard has been initiated.

5.   As far as the question of price control is concerned, the span of control has been gradually reduced since 1979. Presently, under DPCO, 1995 there are 74 bulk drugs and their formulations under price control covering approximately 40% of the total market. The functioning of the Drugs (Price Control) Order, 1995, has brought to light some problems in the administration of the price control mechanism for drugs and pharmaceuticals. In order to review the current drug price control mechanism, with the objective, inter-

alia, of reducing the rigours of price control, where they have become counter-productive, a committee, called the Drugs Price Control Review Committee (DPCRC), under the Chairmanship of Secretary, Department of Chemicals & Petrochemicals was set up in 1999, which has given its report. The recommendations of DPCRC have been examined and taken into account while formulating the "Pharmaceutical Policy – 2002".

6. It has emerged that the domestic drugs and pharmaceuticals industry needs reorientation in order to meet the challenges and harness opportunities arising out of the liberalization of the economy and the impending advent of the product patent regime. It has been decided that the span of price control over drugs and pharmaceuticals would be reduced substantially. However, keeping in view the interest of the weaker sections of the society, it is proposed that the Government will retain the power to intervene comprehensively in cases where prices behave abnormally.

In view of the steps already taken and in the light of the approach indicated in the foregoing paragraphs, the decisions of the Government are detailed below: -

Industrial Licensing

Industrial licensing for all bulk drugs cleared by Drug Controller General (India), all their intermediates and formulations will be abolished, subject to stipulations laid down from time to time in the Industrial Policy, except in the cases of

a) Bulk drugs produced by the use of recombinant DNA technology.

b) Bulk drugs requiring in-vivo use of nucleic acids as the active principles, and

c) Specific cell/tissue targeted formulations.

Foreign Investment

Foreign investment upto 100% will be permitted, subject to stipulations laid down from time to time in the Industrial Policy, through the automatic route in the case of all bulk drugs cleared by Drug Controller

General (India), all their intermediates and formulations, except those, referred to in paragraph above, kept under industrial licensing.

Foreign Technology Agreements

Automatic approval for Foreign Technology Agreements will be available in the case of all bulk drugs cleared by Drug Controller General (India), all their intermediates and formulations, except those referred to in paragraph above, kept under industrial licensing for which a special procedure prescribed by the Government would be followed.

Imports

Imports of drugs and pharmaceuticals will be as per EXIM policy in force. A centralized system of registration will be introduced under the Drugs and Cosmetics Act and Rules made thereunder Ministry of Health and Family Welfare will enforce strict regulatory processes for import of bulk drugs and formulations.

Encouragement to Research and Development (R&D)

a) In principle approval to the establishment of the Pharmaceutical Research and Development Support Fund (PRDSF) under the administrative control of the Department of Science and technology, which will also constitute a Drug Development Promotion Board (DDPB) on the lines of the Technology Development Board to administer the utilization of the PRDSF?

b) With a view to encouraging generation of intellectual property and facilitating indigenous endeavours in pharma R&D, appropriate fiscal incentives would be provided.

Pricing

1. Span of Price Control

The guiding principle for identification of specific bulk drugs for price regulations should continue, as per DPCRC's recommendation, to be:

a) Mass consumption nature of the drug and

b) Absence of sufficient competition in such drugs.

However, the DPCRC's recommendation regarding the new criteria for ascertaining the mass consumption nature of a bulk drug on the basis of the top selling brand is not acceptable as it gives rise to anomalies.

In this context, it may be noted that there is no tailor made data available for the purpose of ascertaining the mass consumption nature and absence of sufficient competition with reference to a particular bulk drug. There is only one source namely, "Retail Store Audit for Pharmaceutical Market in India" published by ORG-MARG, which lists out all major brands and their sale estimates on All India basis. This publication contains data for single ingredient as well as multi-ingredient formulations. However, it does not give complete description of all the ingredients of the pharmaceutical product listed therein.

Hence, there is need to obtain information in regard to composition of each brand, dosage form wise and pack wise, from various other publications /sources Viz.,

a)   Indian Pharmaceutical Guide (IPG)

b)   Current Index of Medical Specialities (CIMS).

c)   Monthly index of Medical Specialities (MIMS).

d)   Drug Today

e)   Information provided by some manufacturers.

f)   Label composition as indicated on market samples.

Though none of these sources can be said to be exhaustive and comprehensive in regard to market information, yet under the given circumstances, these are the best available. It has also been noted that the sale value of any combination formulation is not direct ly relatable to a single particular bulk drug forming part of the combination formulation. Combination formulations involve too many variables, viz., strength of a particular bulk drug and its proportion with respect to other bulk drugs used in the combination formulation, price difference between bulk drugs used in combination formulation; pack sizes, dosage forms etc. In view of these facts, ORG-MARG sales data for combination formulations does not yield information in regard to mass consumption nature and absence of sufficient competition with reference to a particular bulk drug. Also, it is to be borne in mind that processing of such data, which requires cross-checking with other publications and sources of information in regard to composition of each brand, dosage form-wise and pack–wise may involve instances of omission / commission.

In view of above, it would be logical to conclude that although ORG-MARG sale estimates available in regard to all single-ingredient formulations of a particular bulk drug would not yield the sale value of that bulk drug in the form of all its formulations, yet it would adequately reflect the mass consumption nature of that bulk drug in the form of single ingredient formulations, which may be used as a practical indicator for formulating the policy.

The Department through NPPA, with the help of NIPER has developed the desired database for single ingredient formulations from the retail store audit data as published by ORG-MARG. On this basis, the Department proposes to undertake the exercise of identifying the bulk drugs of mass consumption nature and having absence of sufficient competition according to the following methodology: -

i.   The 279 items appearing in the alphabetical lists of Essential Drugs in the National Essential Drug List (1996) of the Ministry of Health and Family Welfare and the 173 items, which are considered important by that Ministry from the point of view of their use in various Health Programmes, in emergency care etc., with the exclusion, as in the past, thereform of sera & vaccines, blood products, combinations etc. should form the total basket out of which selection of bulk drugs be made for price regulation.

ii.   The ORG-MARG data of March 2001 would form the basis for determining the span of price control as suggested by DPCRC.

iii.   The Moving Annual Total (MAT) value for any formulator in respect of any bulk drug will be arrived at by adding the MAT values of all his single-ingredient formulations of that bulk drug, its salts, esters, stereo-isomers and derivatives, coving all the strengths, dosage forms and pack sizes listed against that formulator in all groups

/ categories of the OR-MARG (March 2001).

iv.   The MAT value for all the formulators, as defined in sub-para (iii) above, in respect of a particular bulk drug will be added to arrive at the total MAT value in the retail trade.

v.   The MAT value for an individual formulator, in respect of any bulk drug, as arrived at in sub-para (iii) above, will be the basis for calculating the percentage share of that formulator in the total MAT value arrived at as in sub-para (iv) above, in respect of that bulk drug.

vi.   Bulk Drugs will be kept under price regulation if: -

•   The total MAT value, arrived at as in sub-para (iv) above, in respect of any particular bulk drug is more than Rs.2500 lakhs (Rs. 25 Crores) and the percentage share, as defined in sub-para (v) above, of any of the formulators is 50% or more.

•   The total MAT value, arrived at as in sub-para (iv) above, in respect of any particular bulk drug is less than Rs.2500 lakhs (Rs.25 Crores) but more than Rs.1000 lakhs (Rs.10 Crore) and the percentage share, as defined in sub-para (vi) above, of any of the formulators is 90% or more.

vii.   All formulations containing a bulk drug as identified above, either individually or in combination with other bulk drugs, including those not identified for price control as bulk drug, will be under price control. The Government shall, however, retain the following over-riding power: -

a)   In cases of drugs / formulations listed by the Ministry of Health and Family Welfare, mentioned in sub-paragraph (i) above, and those presently under price control, having significant MAT value as per ORG-MARG but not covered under the criteria in sub-para (vi) above, as a result of this proposal, the NPPA would specially monitor intensively their price movement and consumption pattern. If any unusual movement of prices is observed or brought to the notice of the NPPA, the Authority would work out the price in accordance with the relevant provisions of the price control order.

b)   Maximum Allowable Post-manufacturing Expenses (MAPE) Maximum Allowable Post-manufacturing Expenses (MAPE) will be 100% for indigenously manufactured formulations.

c)   Margin for Imported Formulations

d)   For imported formulations the margin to cover selling and distribution expenses including interest and importer's profit shall not exceed fifty percent of the landed cost.

2.   Pricing of Formulations:

i.   For Scheduled formulations, prices shall be determined as per the present practice. The time frame for granting price approvals will be two months from the date of the receipt of the complete prescribed information.

ii.   The present stipulation that a manufacturer, distributor or wholesaler shall sell a formulation to a retailer, unless otherwise permitted under the provisions of Drugs (Prices Control) Order or any other order made thereunder, at a price equal to the retail price, as specified by an order or notified by the Government, (excluding excise duty, if any) minus sixteen percent thereof in case of Scheduled drugs, will continue.

iii.   The present provision of limiting profitability of pharmaceutical companies, as per the Third Schedule of the present Drugs (Prices Control) Order, 1995, would be done away with. However, if necessary so to do in public interest, price of any formulation including a non-Scheduled formulation would be fixed or revised by the Government.

3.   Ceiling prices:

Ceiling prices may be fixed for any formulation, from time to time, and it would be obligatory for all, including small-scale units or those marketing under generic name, to follow the price so fixed.

4.   Exemptions:

i.   A manufacturer producing a new drug patented under the Indian Paten Act, 1970, and not produced elsewhere, if developed through indigenous R&D, would be eligible for exemption from price control in respect of that drug for a period of 15 years from the date of the commencement of its commercial production in the country.

ii.   A manufacturer producing a drug in the country by a process developed through indigenous R&D and patented under the Indian Patent Act, 1970, would be eligible for exemption from price control in respect of that drug till the expiry of the patent from the date of the commencement of its commercial production in the country by the new patented process.

iii.   A formulation involving a new delivery system developed through   indigenous R&D and patented under the Indian Patent Act, 1970, for process patent for formulation involving new delivery system would be eligible for exemption from price control in favour of the patent holder formulator from the date of the commencement of its commercial production in the country till the expiry of the patent.

iv.   The DPCRC has suggested that the low cost drugs measured in terms of "cost per day per medicine" may be taken out of price control. Any formulator can represent to NPPA with proof of per day cost to consumer-patient. NPPA will be authorized to exempt such formulation from price control if its cost to consumer-patient does not exceed Rs.2/- per day, under intimation to the Government. All orders passed by the NPPA will be prospective in operation. Whenever the concerned formulator wishes to revise the price, he, before effecting any change in price, would be bound to inform NPPA and seek fresh exemption and in case the cost to consumer-patient, on the basis of the proposed revised price, exceeds beyond the limit of Rs.2/- per day, obtain the necessary price approval.

5.   Pricing of Scheduled Bulk Drugs

i.   For a Scheduled bulk drug, the rate of return in case of basic manufacture would be higher by 4 per cent over the existing 14 per cent on et worth or 22 per cent on capital employed. The time frame for granting price approvals will be 4 months from the date of receipt of the complete prescribed information.

ii.   The Government shall, however, retain the overriding power of fixing the maximum sale price of any bulk drug, in public interest.

6.   Monitoring:

i.   The DPCRC's recommendations to have effective monitoring and enforcement system and to move away from the "controlled regime" to a recommendation as imports will increasingly compete with local drugs and pharmaceuticals in the domestic market. A new system based on solely market prices data is required to be evolved and controls applied selectively only to cases where, either profiteering or monopoly profit seeking is noticed. The National Pharmaceutical Pricing Authority, set up in August, 1997, would need to be revamped and reoriented for this purpose. It will continue to be entrusted with the task of price fixation / price revision and other related matters, and would be empowered to take final decisions. It would also monitor the prices of decontrolled drugs and formulations and over-see the implementation of the drug prices control orders.

ii.   The Government would have the power of review of the price fixation / and price revision orders / notifications of NPPA.

iii.   Although the prices of some bulk drugs have been steadily decreasing, yet the same do not get reflected in the retail price of non-Scheduled formulations. Also, there is need to check high margin/commission offered to the trade by printing high prices on the labels of medicines to the detriment of the consumers. IT is, therefore, proposed to strengthen the National Pharmaceutical Pricing Authority by providing appropriate powers under the DPCO which would make it mandatory for the manufacturer to furnish all information as called for by NPPA and also to regulate such prices, wherever, required.

iv.   The other recommendations of DPCRC like giving powers to drug control authorities to dispose of small and petty offences etc., will required an amendment to the Essential Commodities

Act. This suggestion is considered not practicable. Monitoring price movement of drugs sold in the country as well as that of imported formulations will require developing appropriate mechanism in the NPPA.

7. Drug Price Equalization Account (DPEA):

Provision would be made in the new Drugs (Prices Control) Order (DPCO) to ensure that amounts which have already accrued to the DPEA and those which are likely to accrue as a result of action in the past, are protected and used for the purpose stipulated in the existing DPCO.

QUALITY ASPECTS

The Ministry of Health & Family Welfare would:

i. Progressively benchmark the regulatory standards against the international standards for manufacturing.

ii. Progressively harmonize standards for clinical testing with international practices.

iii. Streamline the procedures and steps for quick evaluation and clearance of new drug applications, developed in India through indigenous R&D, and

iv. Set up a world class Central Drug Standard Control Organization (CDSCO) by modernizing, restructuring and reforming the existing system and establish an effective net work of drugs standards enforcement administrations in the States with the CDSCO as a nodal centre, to ensure high standards of quality, safety and efficacy of drugs and pharmaceuticals.

PHARMA EDUCATION AND TRAINING

The National Institute of Pharmaceutical Education and Research (NIPER) has been set up by the Government of India as an institute of "national importance" to achieve excellence in pharmaceutical sciences and technologies, education and training. Through this institute, Government's endeavour will be to upgrade the standards of pharmacy education and R&D. Besides tackling problems of human resources development for academia and the indigenous pharmaceutical industry, the institute will make efforts to maximize collaborative research with the industry and other technical institutes in the area of drug discovery and pharma technology development.

ESSAY QUESTIONS

1. Write a note on Establishment, Constitution and Functions of Animal Welfare Board of India.

2. Write a note on Cruelty of Animal.

3. How does the Prevention of Cruelty to Animal Act 1960 control the performance of experiments on animals?

4. Write a note on Licensing Procedure under Factories Act 1948.

5. Write a note on provision of Health and Safety as under Factories Act 1948.

6. What do you mean by GATT? Write a note on Tokyo round and progress of GATT.

7. What do you mean by WTO? Write a note on WTO.

8. Differentiate between GATT and WTO.

9. Write a note on procedure for Application for Patent.

10. Write a note on objectives of Pharmaceutical Policy Act 2002.

11. What are the provisions provided for pricing under Pharmaceutical policy 2002?

12. What are provisions related to Quality Aspects and Pharmacy Education and Training under Pharmaceutical policy 2002?

SHORT QUESTIONS

1. What are the objectives of Prevention of Cruelty to Animal Act 1960.

2. Define.

    a)   Captive animal.

    b)   Domestic animal.

    c)   Breeder.

    d)   Establishment.

    e)   Experiment.

3. Define.

    a)   Commercial establishment.

    b)   Establishment.

    c)   Shop.

    d)   Wages.

4 What are the provisions for Registration of Establishment under AP State Shops and Establishment Act 1988?

5 What are provisions provided by AP State Shops and Establishment Act 1988 regarding Hours of working, Opening/closing times and Closing days?

6 Write a note on Cleanliness/Ventilation/Lighting as under the provision of the AP State Shops and Establishment Act 1988.

7 Write a note on Employment of Women and Children under the provision of AP State Shops and Establishment Act 1988.

8 What are the provisions provided for health and safety under AP State Shops and Establishment Act 1988?

9 Write a note on appointment, powers and duties of Chief Inspector.

10 What are the objectives of Factory Act 1948?

11 Define.

    a)   Competent person.

    b)   Hazardous processes.

    c)   Workers.

    d)   Factory.

    e)   Occupier.

12   Define.

    a)   Exclusive licence.

    b)   Invention.

    c)   Patents.

    d)   True or first inventor.

13   Write a note on Exclusive Marketing Rights.

14   Write a note on Registration of Patents.

15   Write a note on Inventions not patentable.